WOODY GUTHRIE'S

Wardy forty

GREYSTONE PARK STATE HOSPITAL REVISITED

by Phillip Buehler

In collaboration with Nora Guthrie and the Woody Guthrie Archives

Edited and designed by Steven Brower

Woody Guthrie Publications, Inc.

I've photographed abandoned spaces for over thirty years, starting with a trip to Ellis Island in a rowboat while I was still in high school. I've learned you never know what you'll find inside, but I had no idea that I'd find photographs of Woody Guthrie when I climbed into a broken window at Greystone Park State Hospital. Or that I'd spend the next ten years talking to people who knew him, photographing the abandoned buildings, and digging through the Woody Guthrie Archives. This is the story Woody left behind.–*Phillip Buehler*

I got a phone call in the office from the state troopers in New Jersey. They got the number, Woody told them to call. And they explained that he was picked up for being a vagrant: "Is that so?" I said, "No, he's not a vagrant." And he'd said that he's sick, and I said, "That's true, and that should be taken care of from a medical point of view, rather than arrested." I merely certified what Woody was telling them. The result was that he wasn't arrested, but was committed to a hospital.–*Harold Leventhal*

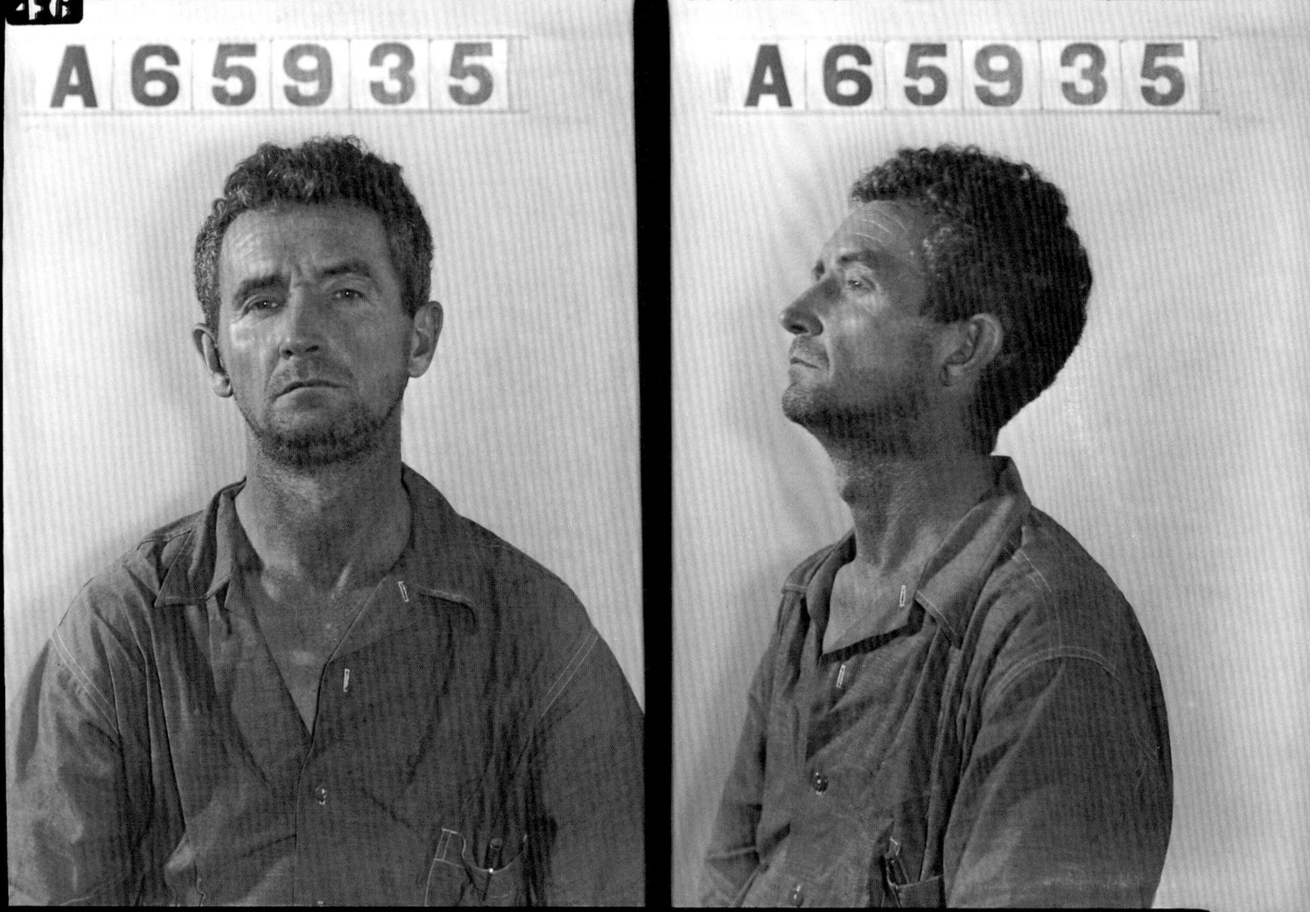
A65935
A65935

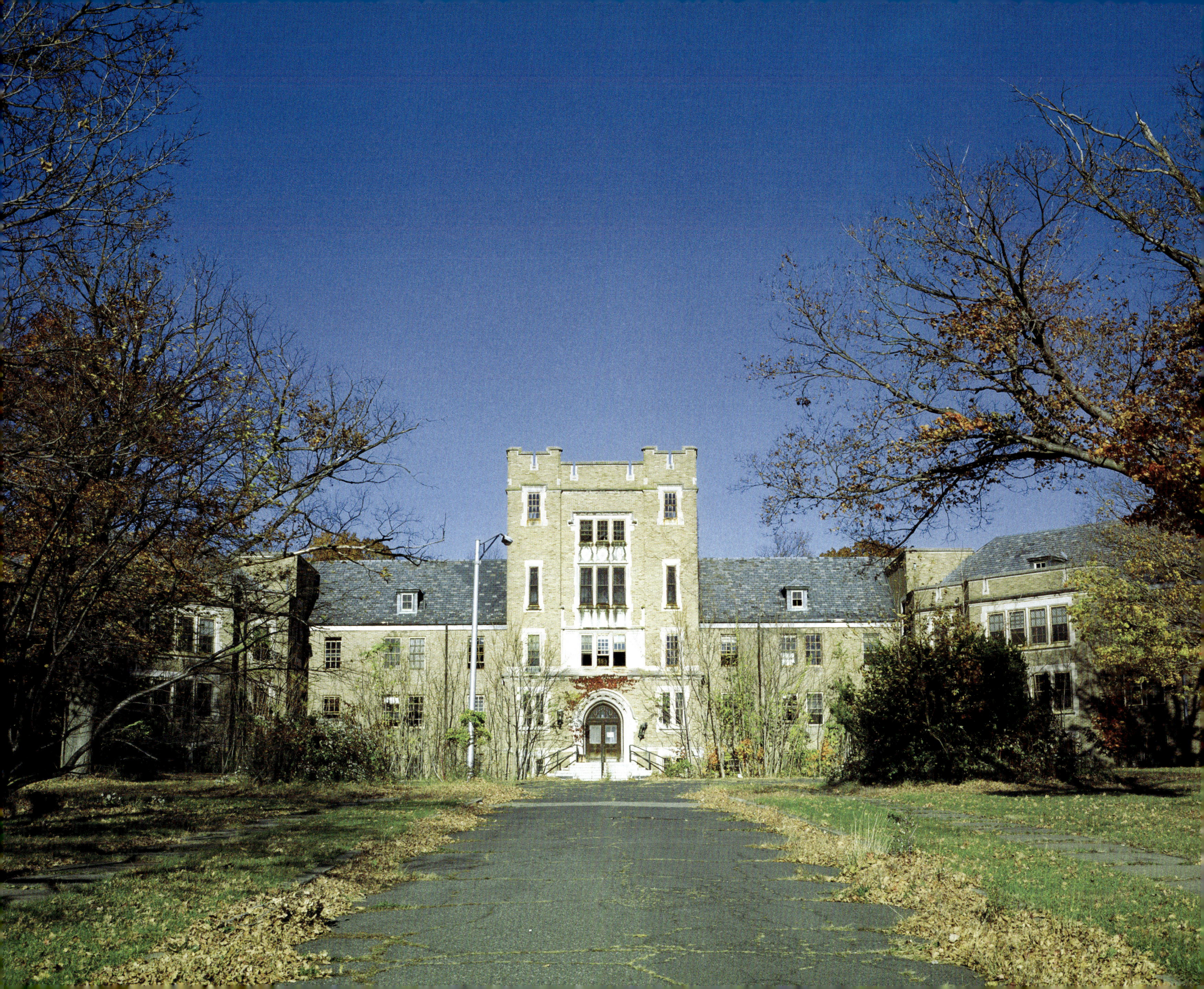

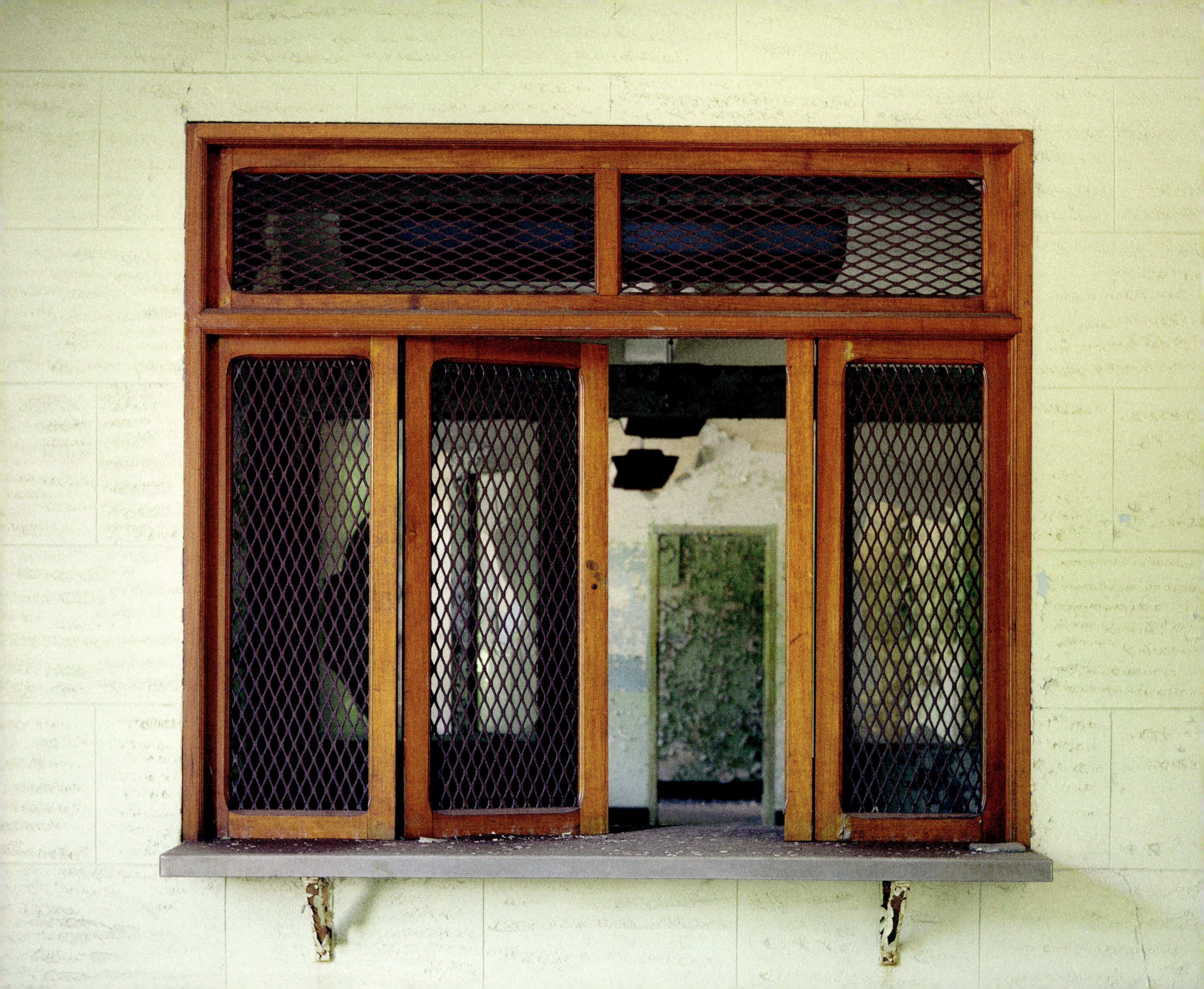

We just were told that he was going to be very sick and that situation was hopeless and helpless. And that everyone advised me to tell the children that their father had died, that they should not see him deteriorate. Everybody, including the doctors. And Woody and I talked it over and I kept saying, "You know, this is crazy." I told Woody we would never eliminate the children from his life, but we were advised that he should go into the hospital and stay there because they thought he was going to be what they call a vegetable at the end of his life. Well, he never was.*–Marjorie Guthrie*

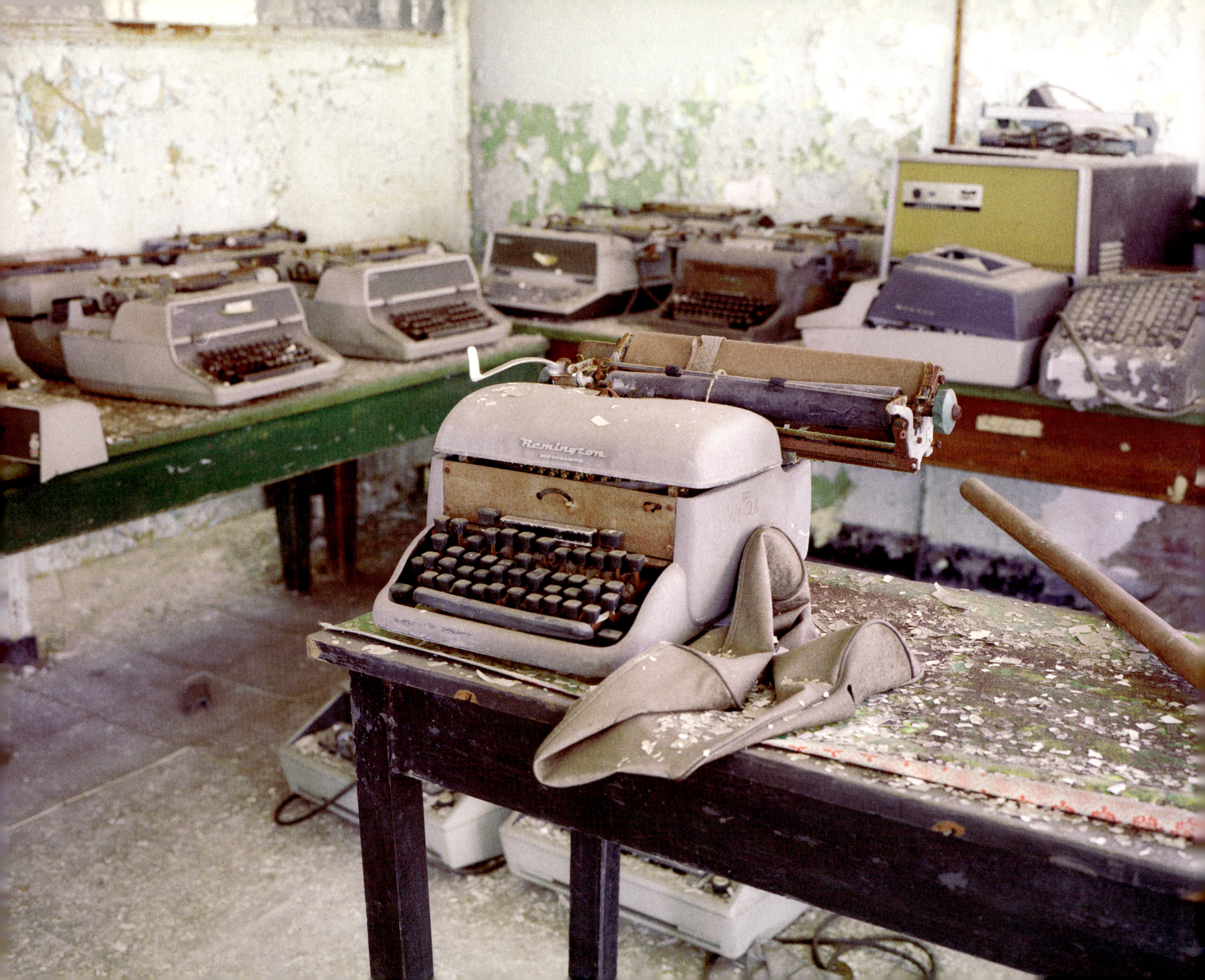
Remington

Name Woodrow Wilson Guthrie Case No. 65935

S U M M A R Y

Admitted: May 29, 1956 **Informant: hospital records**

FAMILY HISTORY: Charles E. Guthrie, father, living, born in United States. Mother Nora B. Tanner, born in United States, deceased.

PERSONAL HISTORY: Patient born in Oklahoma, July 14, 1912, married, last address, 72 Bank Street, Brooklyn, New York.

PERSONALITY: No information available.

ONSET OF PRESENT CONDITION: Abstract from commitment papers states, number of previous attacks, unknown; age at first attack, 42; duration of present attack, 2 years; onset, gradual; physical condition, fair; personal habits, unclean; tendencies, none; supposed cause, unknown. In physician's presence said, "I got $3000 for writing a song. I left Brooklyn State Hospital on May 23, 1956. I wanted to find the orphans to give them the money. I wrote about 8000 songs and I got $10,000 for writing." Untidy, unkempt, kept talking all through interview about all the money he has. Lacks insight and judgement. Grandiose ideas. Untidy and unkempt. Wanders about the highways. Patient was arrested for wandering aimlessly on the highways. Regularly committed to this hospital from Morris County Jail May 29, 1956.

HOSPITAL RESIDENCE (MENTAL): Tendencies were not given; alleged cause, unknown. Overproductive. Emotionally circumstantial, rambling; his answers were only partially relevant; kept talking about something else. TREND: He stated that he has been hearing voices, also saw the persons who have been talking to him, like Jesus and Maria. They have been giving advice to him as to what to do. They calmed him down and told him not to worry about this or that problem. He does not think that people are talking behind his back but if anything is wrong it would not harm him. He has special abilities in music and made some ten thousand dollars in writing songs. He was in the Brooklyn State Hospital for three years and signed himself out about three weeks ago. He wanted to get away from New York because his wife wanted to get a divorce. She is running around with other men. He has a child, age three. It was born shortly before he went to Brooklyn. He claims that he is playing guitars and fiddles in spite of his stiff fingers on the right hand which he burned in 1953. He went as far as the tenth grade in school and was in the Merchant Marine during the war and was in the Air Force for a short while. (There is a question in the mind of the examiner whether all this is fantasy.) He claims that he gets $66 compensation from the government. Throughout the interview he remained manneristic and gesturing in a grandiose way. He also had a silly smile on his face at times. His affect was inappropriate. Sensorium, clear. Correctly oriented in all spheres. Remote and recent past memory good. Intelligence rathing, average. Insight and judgment; insight lacking, judgement defective.

HOSPITAL RESIDENCE (PHYSICAL): This is a 44 year old white man with flat chest, dropped right shoulder and wrist. There is a systolic murmur over his heart area, best audible in left 6th intercostal space 2 fingers medially to nipple line in upright position, after exercise. His liver is enlarged 1 finger below costal margin in nipple line, firm with sharp edge. There is a large recurrent left inguinal hernia, reduceable. Gait is swaying; speech slurred. Pulse rate 80 regular. Blood pressure 110/74. This man is 5' 6" tall; weight 125 pounds. He has brown-grey hair and blue eyes. Laboratory findings negative or within normal limits.

The examining psychiatrist may have been a foreigner or something like that, who knew nothing about Woody Guthrie. He would think he was paranoid for saying he had written an awful lot of songs and so on. That was an admission note, and I'm sure the diagnosis must have been changed later on when it became clear that he had Huntington's Chorea. . . finally they saw the light.–*Dr. Vincenzo Cocilovo*

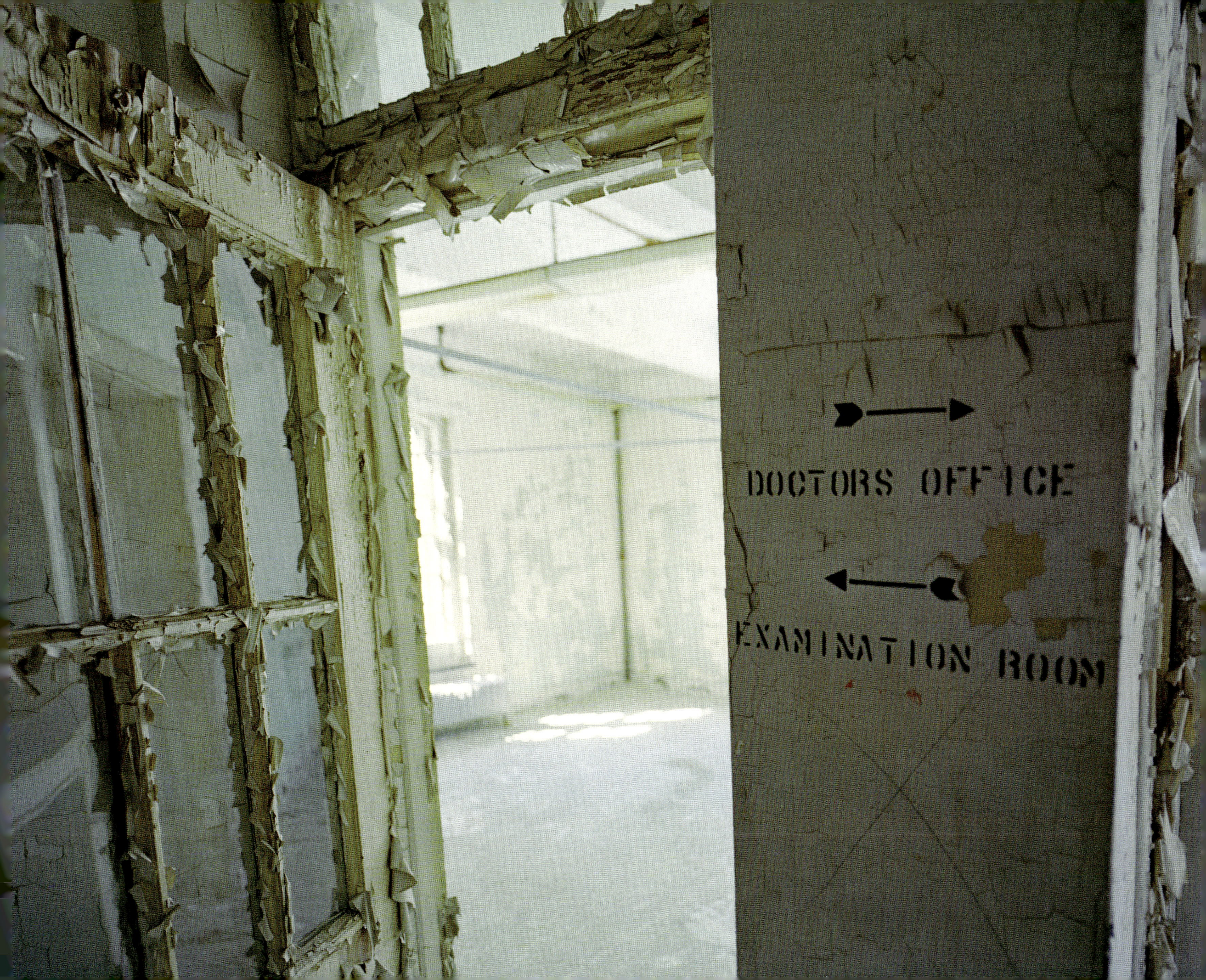
DOCTORS OFFICE
EXAMINATION ROOM

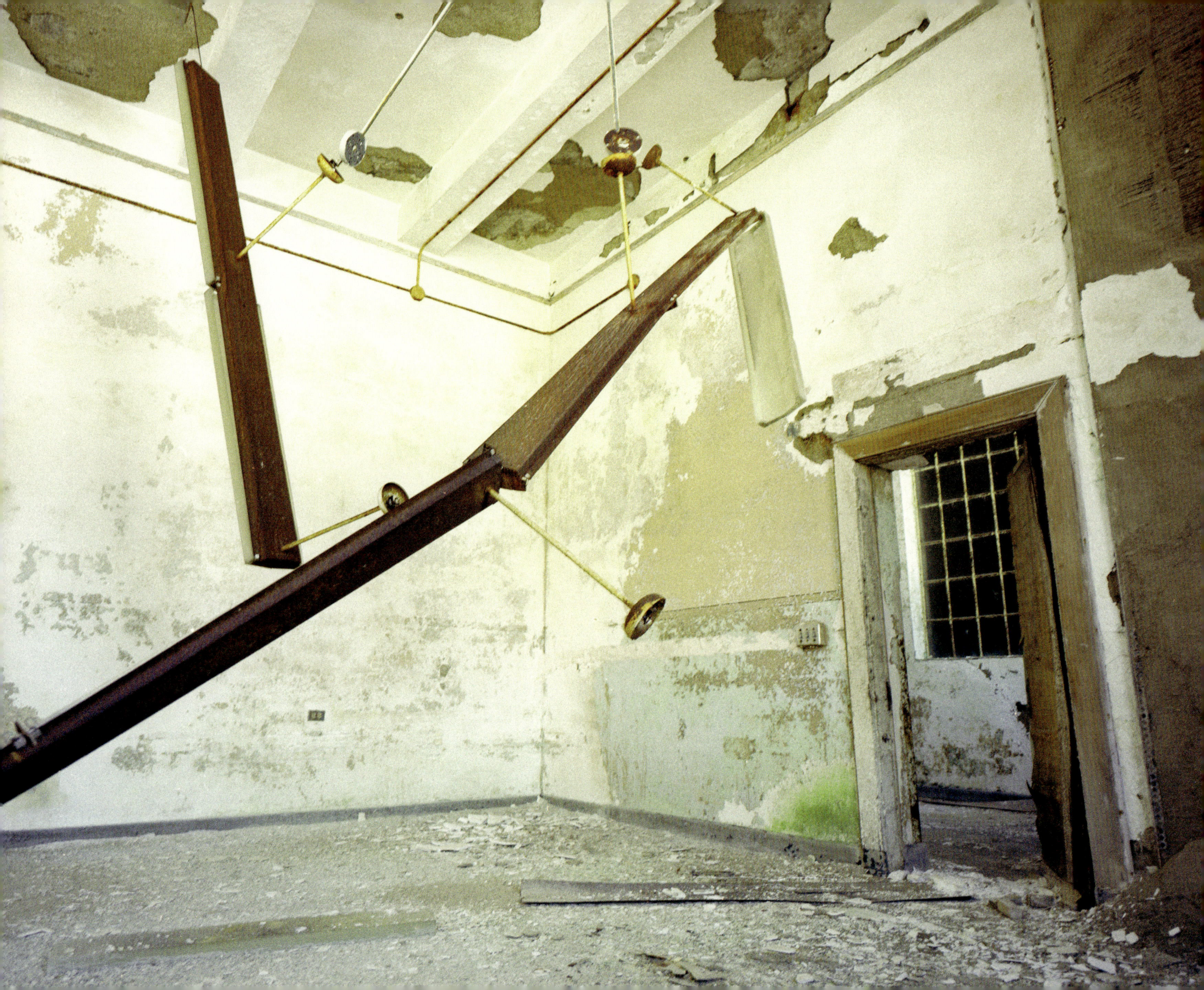

ONDITION: Abstract from

age at first attack,

condition, fair; personal

In physician's presence said,

te Hospital on May 23, 1956.

I wrote about 8000 songs and I got

lking all through interview about all the

Grandiose ideas. Untidy and unkempt.

ested for wandering aimlessly on the highway

l from Morris County Jail May 29, 1956.

Tendencies were not given

I remember my mom was called by a German psychologist who said, "Mrs. Guthrie, your husband is really ill and we're glad they brought him in." She says, "Oh, tell me what's going on?" He said, "Well, first of all, he's got delusions of grandeur. He thinks he's a well-known singer and has written books and people were singing his songs." She said, "What do you mean?" He said, "He thinks he's well known." She said, "He is well known!" They said "Oh." –*Arlo Guthrie*

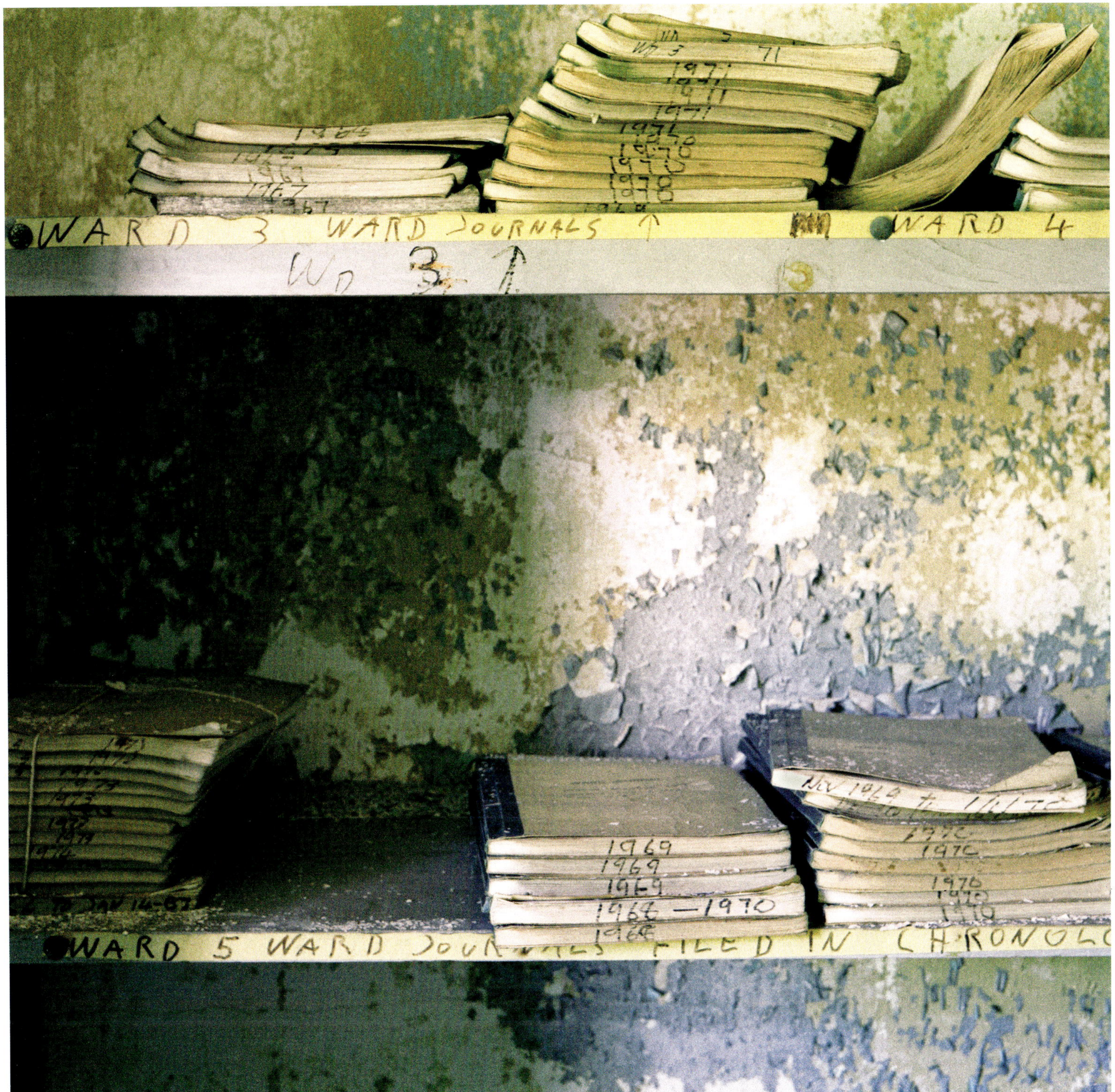
WARD 3 WARD JOURNALS
WARD 4
WARD 5 WARD JOURNALS FILED IN CHRONOL

Marjorie spoke about how he was initially misdiagnosed, that there was so much ignorance that was present.

—Dr. Michael Hayden

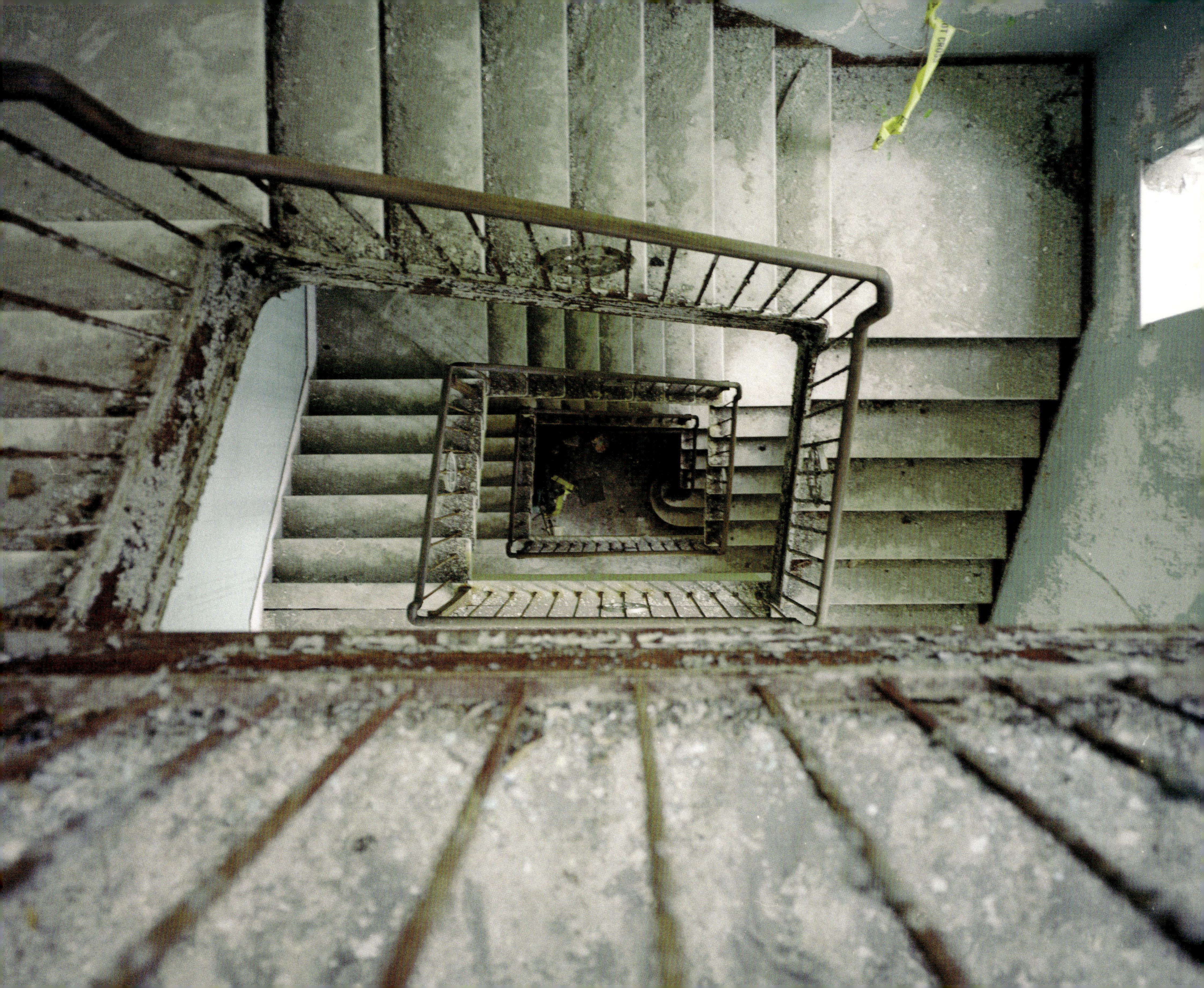

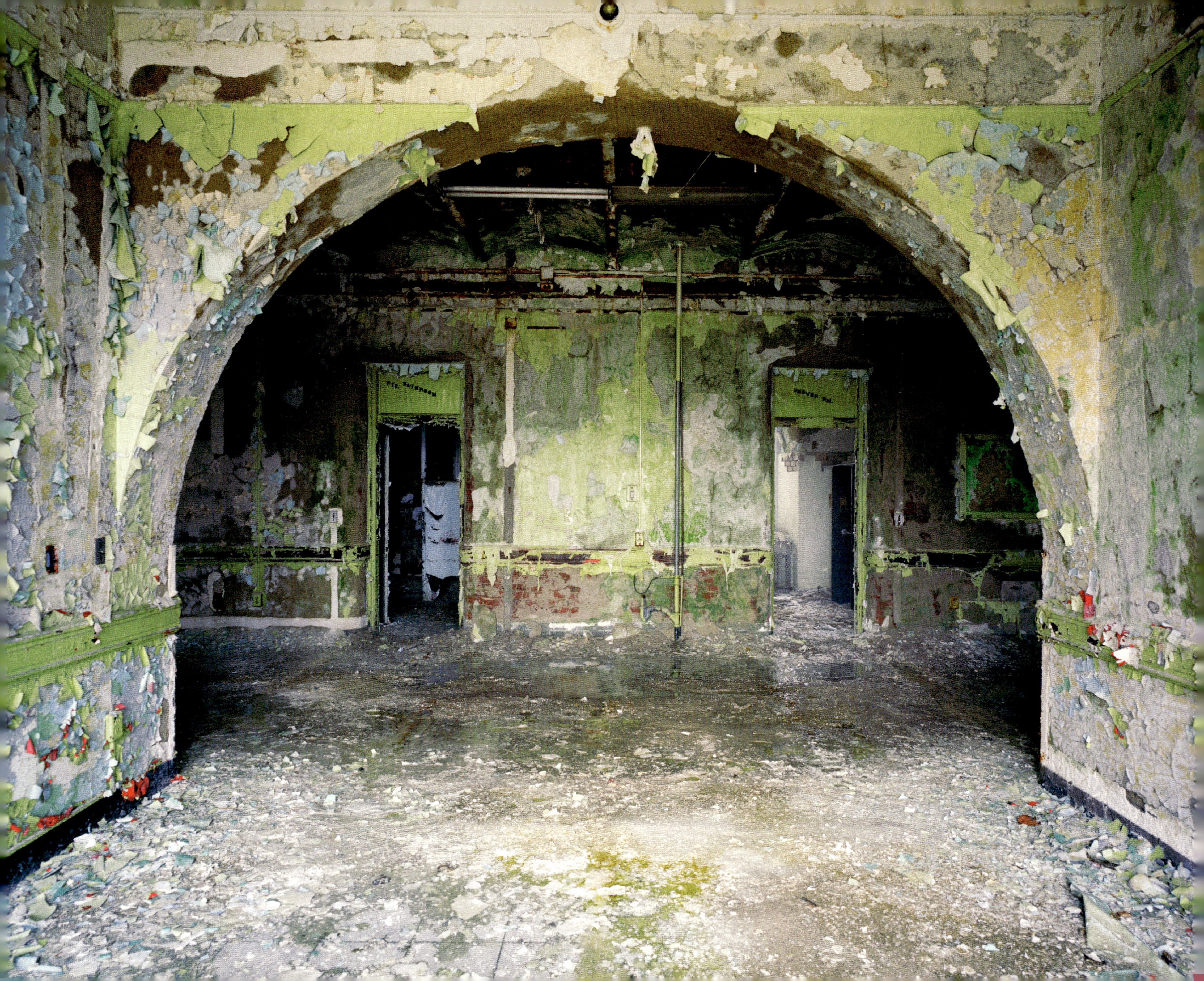
PTS. BATHROOM
SHOWER RM.

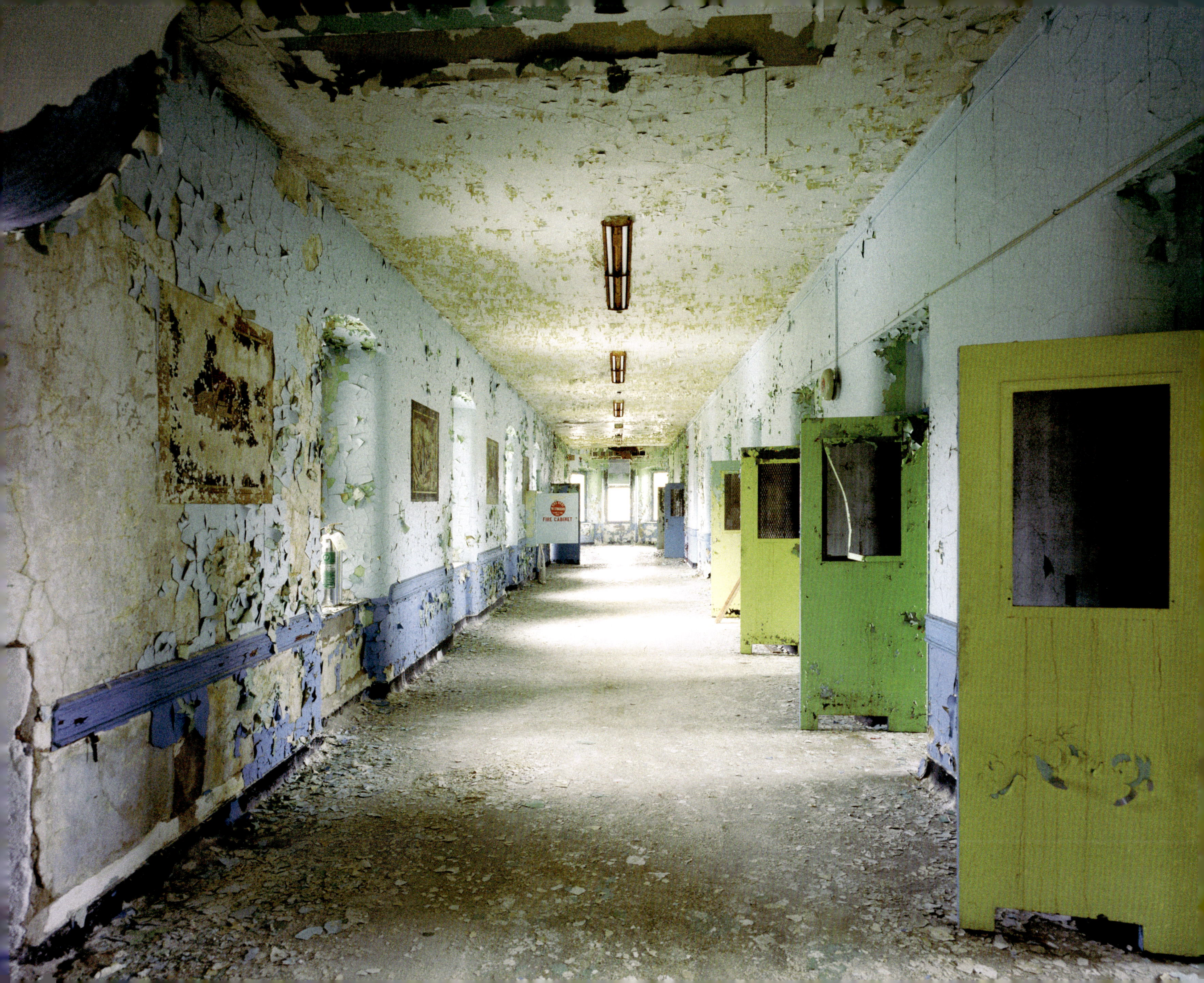
FIRE CABINET

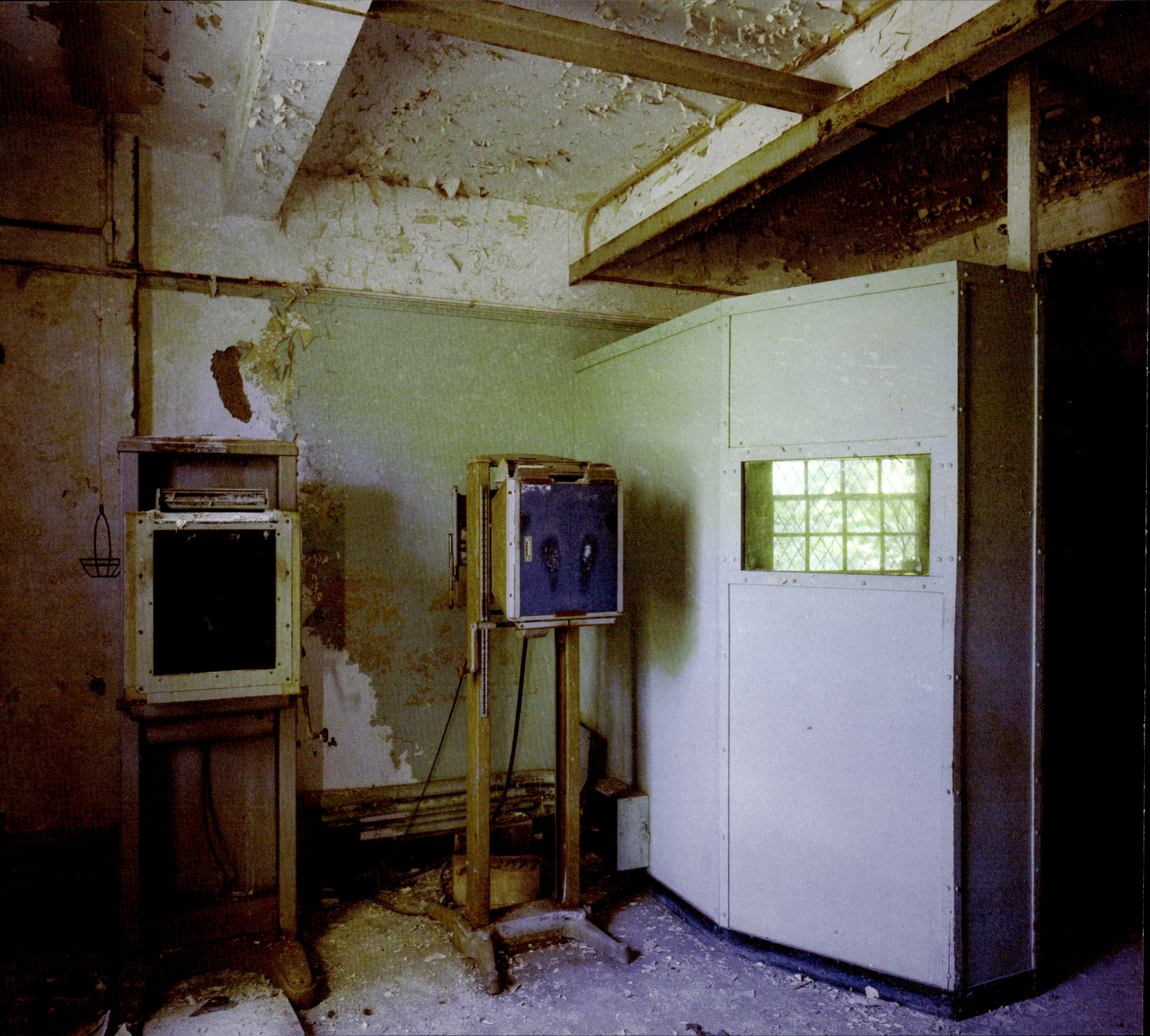

Well, I didn't all of a sudden realize that he had Huntington's Disease. Over the years my mom sort of gradually introduced whatever she knew. Actually, in the beginning, no one knew anything. Even my dad thought that he was suffering from alcoholism, or God knows what. He was convinced he couldn't have the same disease his mom had, because he had some misconceptions about how it was transmitted. And so, little by little, at the insistence of my mom, even the doctors had to learn stuff. She was very wonderful that way. She had some concerns about her kids, obviously, and she really spent a good decade or two discovering what was going on. So there wasn't one moment when I suddenly was told something. It was gradually over years—first we realized our dad was sick, then he had some sort of disorder, and blah blah blah, and, little by little, we sort of knew what was going on.—*Arlo Guthrie*

Dear Mrs. Ladlie;

I regret in the delay in answering your letter of April 12th in reference to Woodrow Wilson Guthrie. I had been out of New York for some weeks.

To the best of my knowledge Mr. Guthrie has never had any permanent established legal residence for a good number of years. He has always drifted from one part of the country to another, staying at various places for indefinite times. Those of us who know him, could never be able to pin him down as to where his official residence was—he never had one as such. I do not believe Mr. Guthrie voted for the past many of years—as he did not stay in one place long enough. One of Mr. Guthrie's problems for (h)is friends has been his constant lust for wandering-that has made him a problem for his friends and family, over the years.

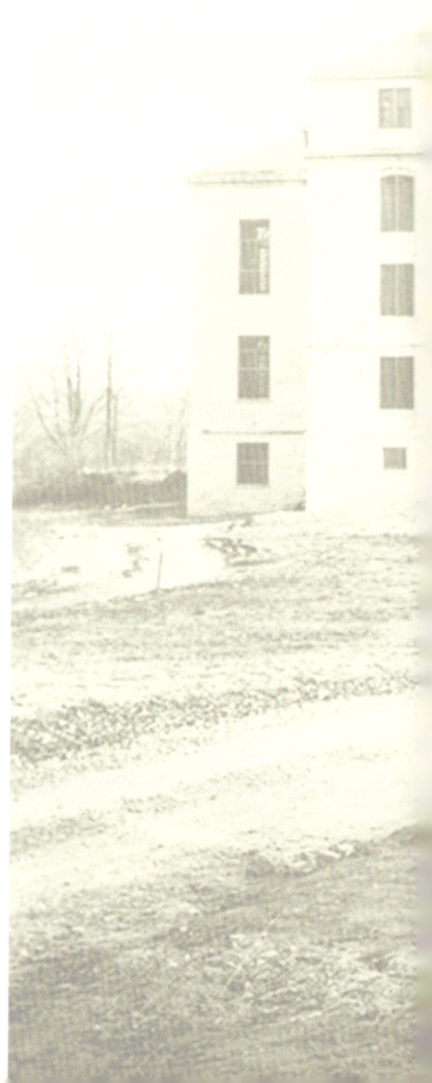

I trust that you (are) aware that some years back Mr. Guthrie was one of America's top folk singer, writer and songwriter–having his own radio show and appearing in the top clubs in the USA. He wrote many famous folk songs, the best known being SO LONG IT'S BEEN GOOD TO KNOW YOU. He has a book published "Bound for Glory" that was a best seller years ago. Unfortunately for the past 8 or more years Mr. Guthrie has not been as consistent as he should. I mention his background to emphasis that he is the kind if person, as a folk artist, who for years has wandered about America.

Very truly yours,
Harold Leventhal

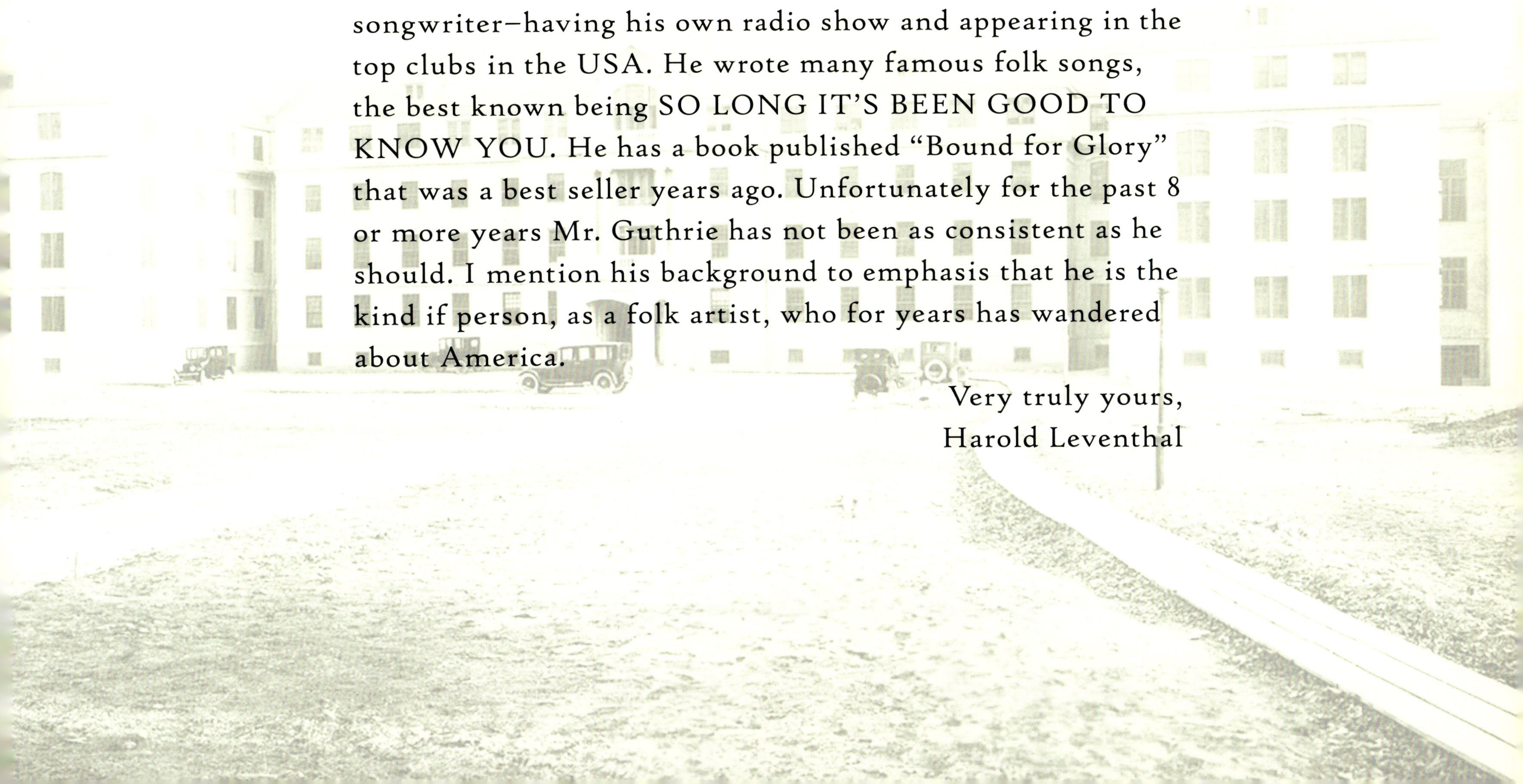

He has been called by many people a great folk artist, in his writings and in his performance, he received mail from people all over the country who liked his songs. He has sung for every major network in the country. I could name prominent people who claim they were inspired by him. The Boy Scouts and Girl Scouts use his songs, the Board of Education in various states use his songs. He has written literally thousands of songs and poems. He has been quoted by many famous writers in their books.

His works are still yet to be published and I and a few interested persons are going ahead with our plans to bring much unpublished material to the readers. It will take time since I am still working regularly and busy raising our family. The writings are no problem since they are all in tangible form. . . it is he, the man that of course is our real problem. What can we do with him? What can you do for him? These are the questions that need answering.

—Marjorie Guthrie, letter to doctors at Greystone Park State Hospital, July 18, 1956.

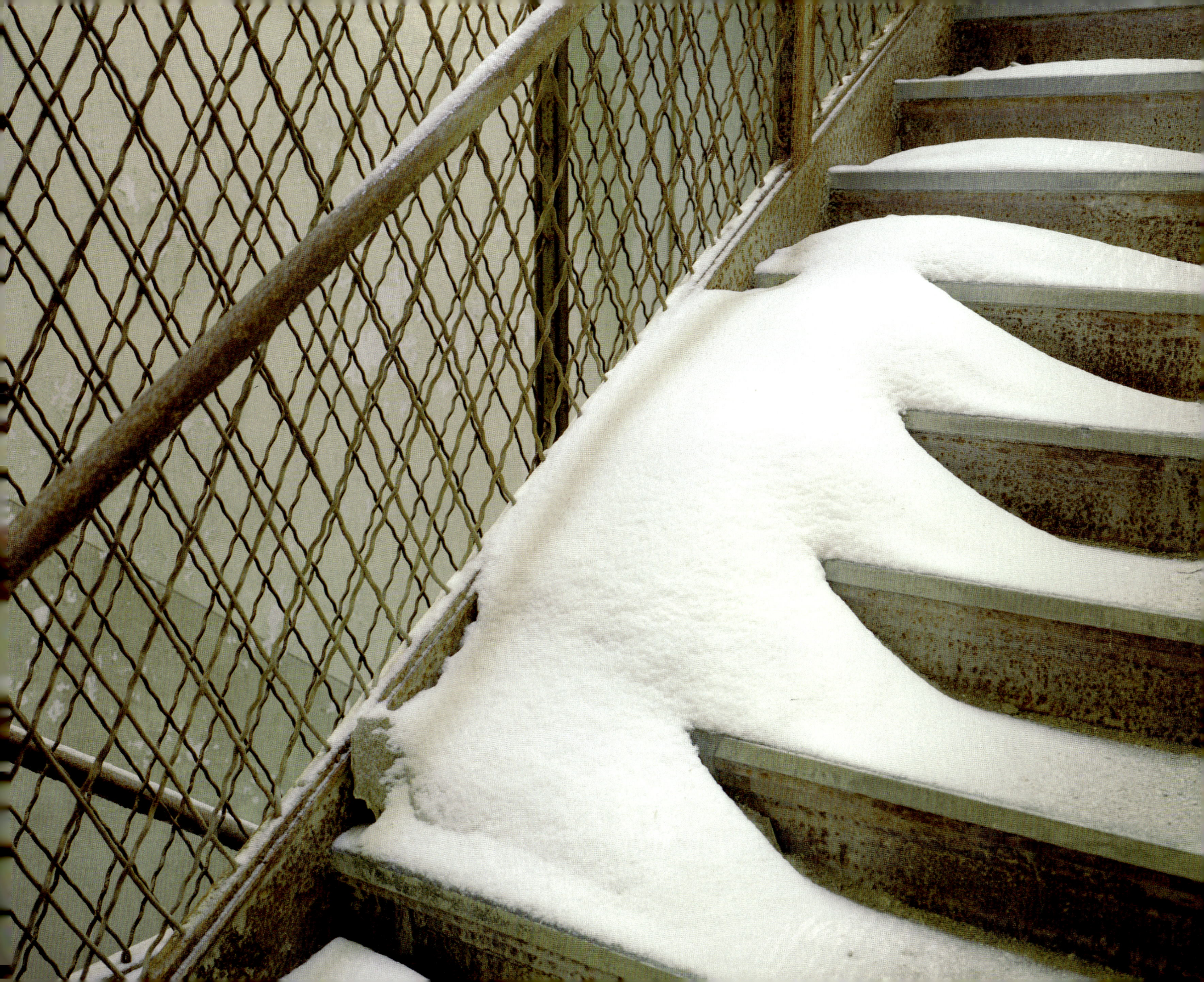

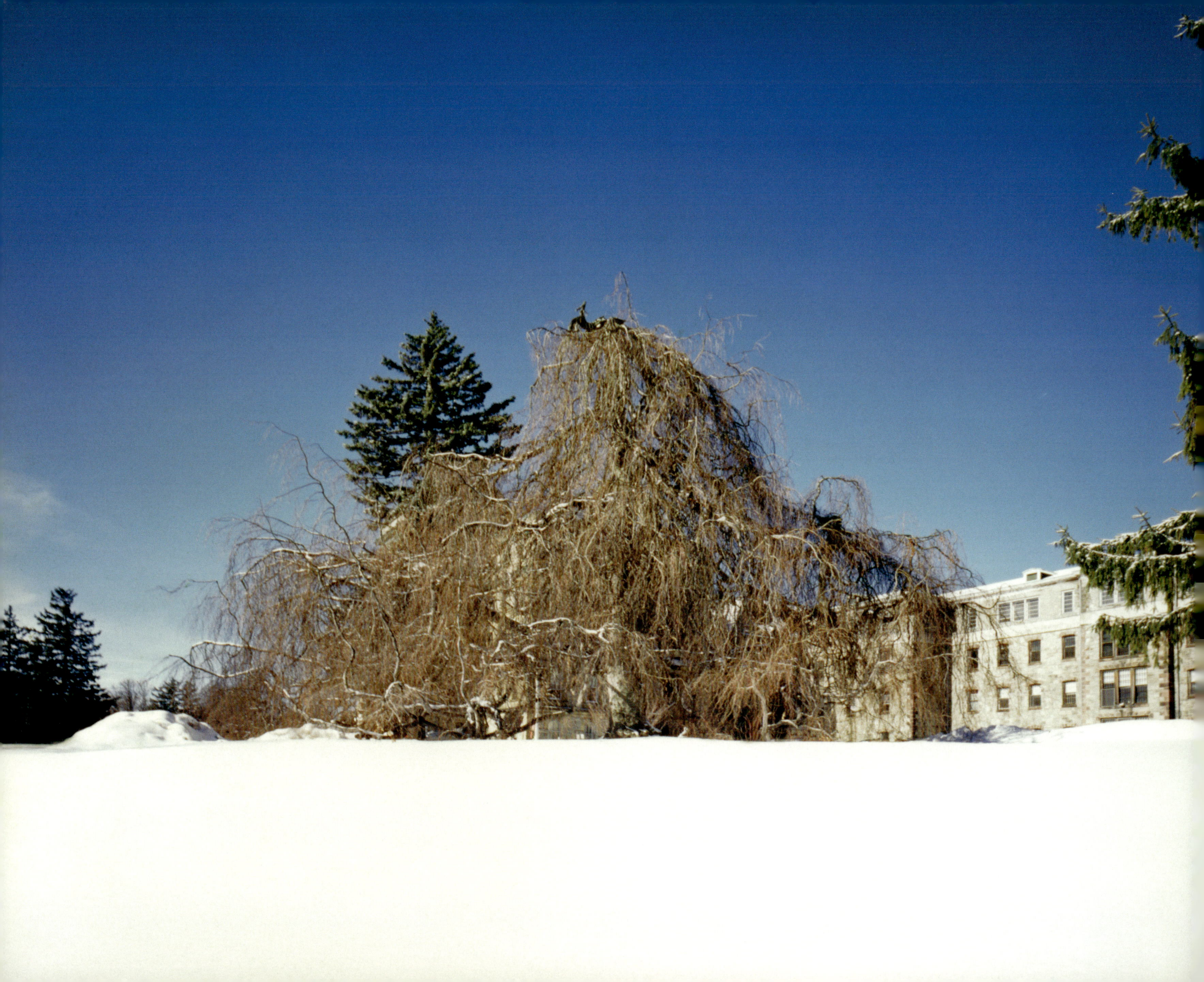

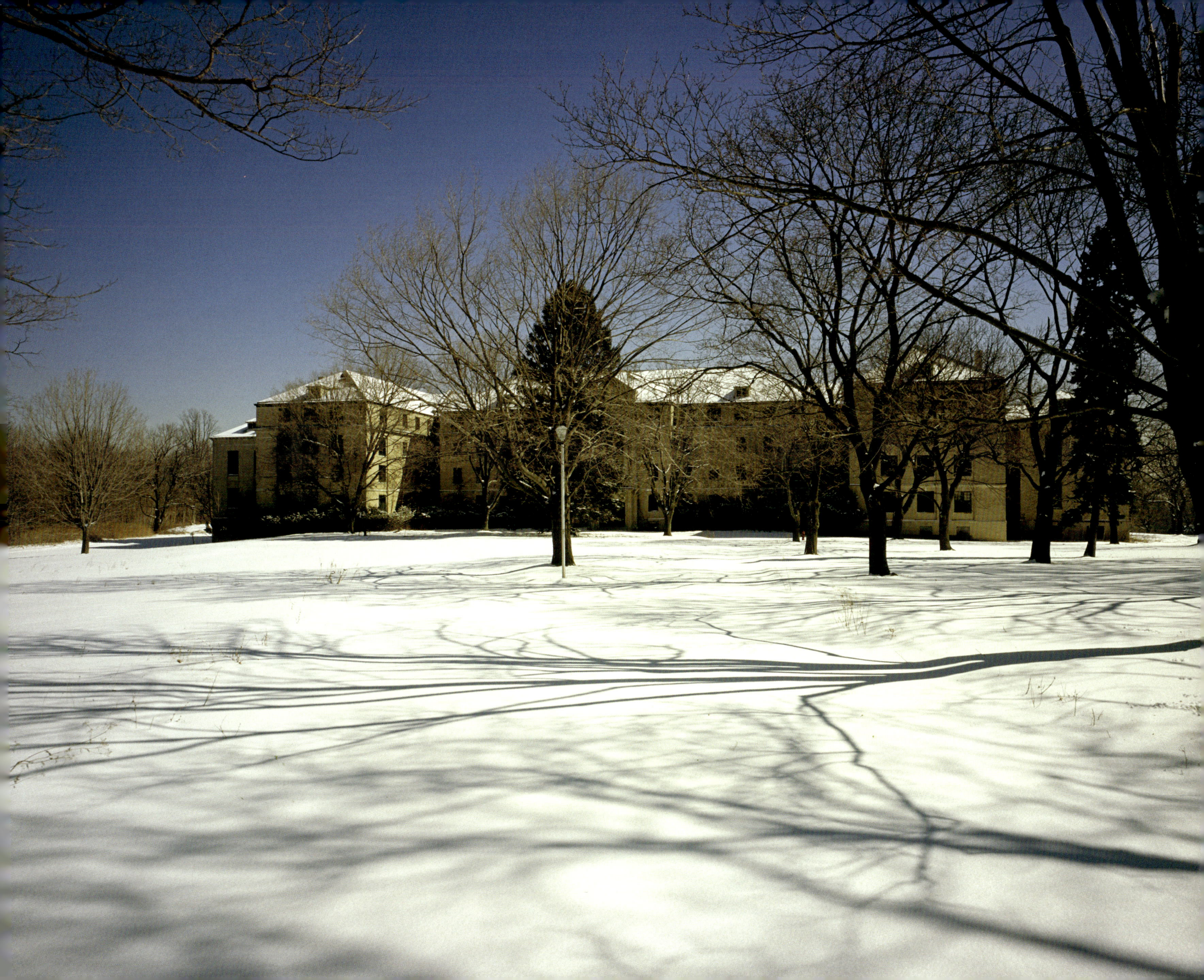

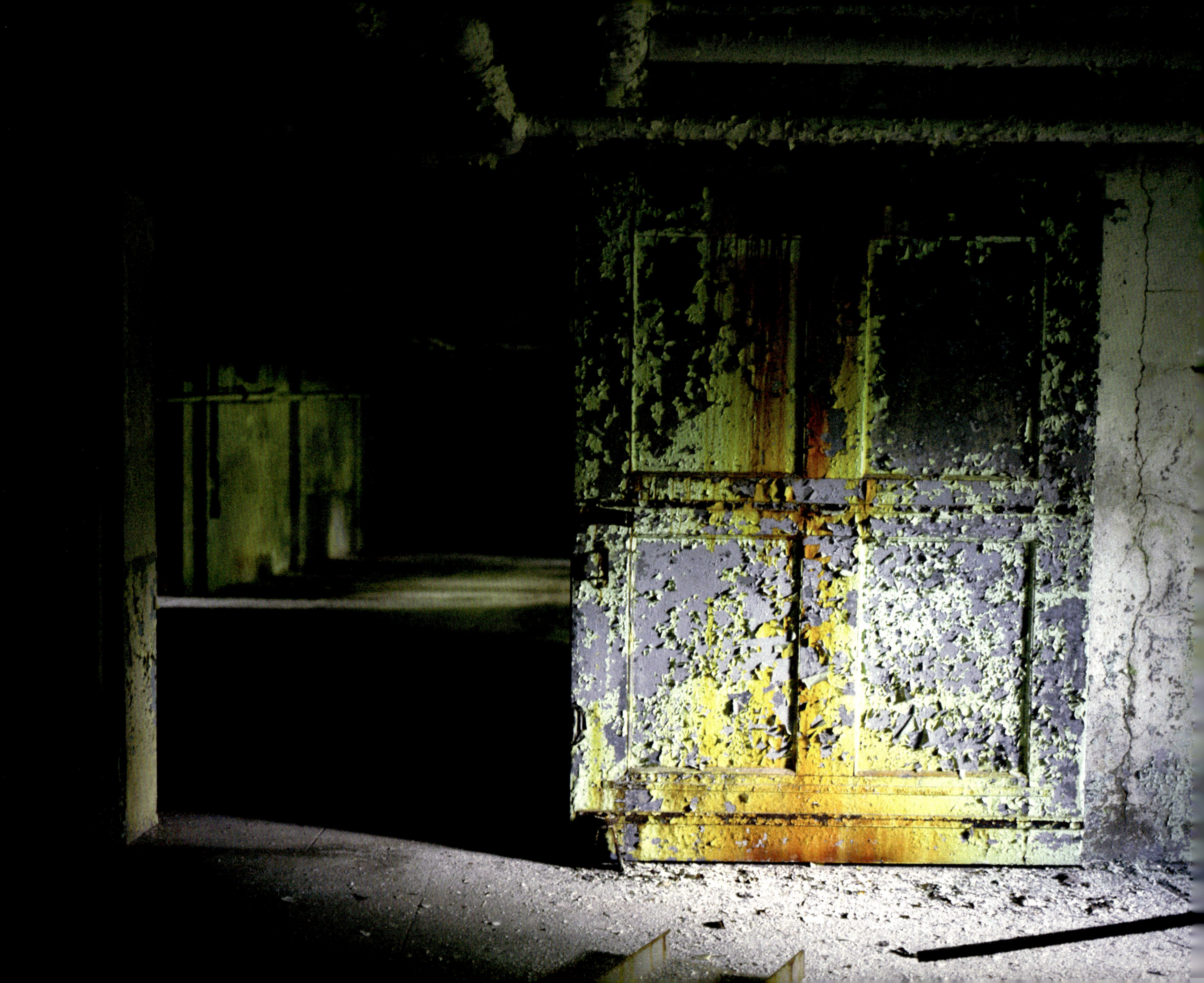

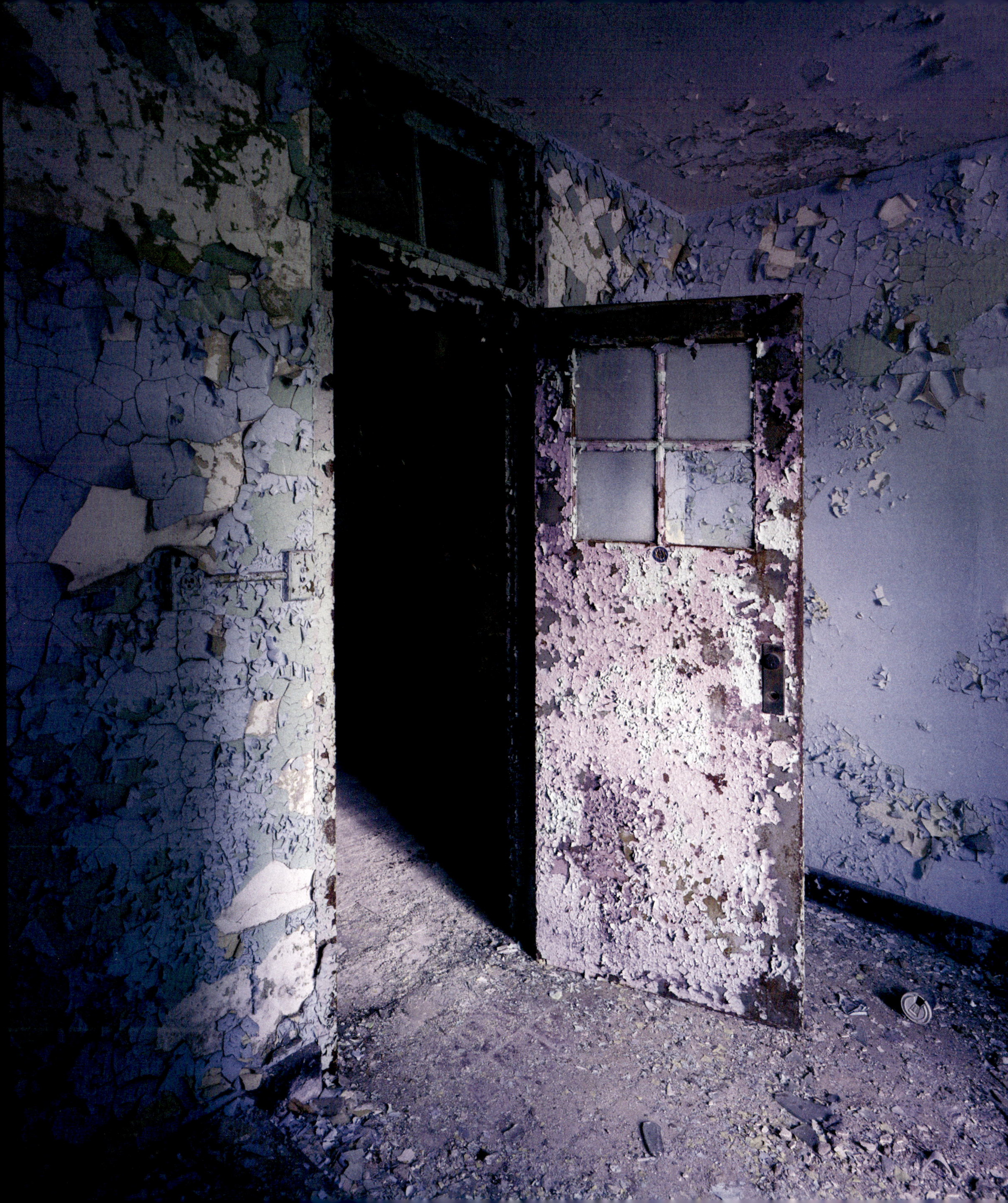

My father lived in a ward with many other patients. I remember one time walking through the entire ward with beds lined on both sides to get to my father's bed at the very end. The walk seemed to take forever. All around us were strange people yelling, talking to themselves, uninhibited or somber. I walked as close to my mother as possible, hiding behind her skirts as she greeted many patients with a cheery and energetic, "hello." I couldn't understand why she wasn't terrified. I was.*–Nora Guthrie*

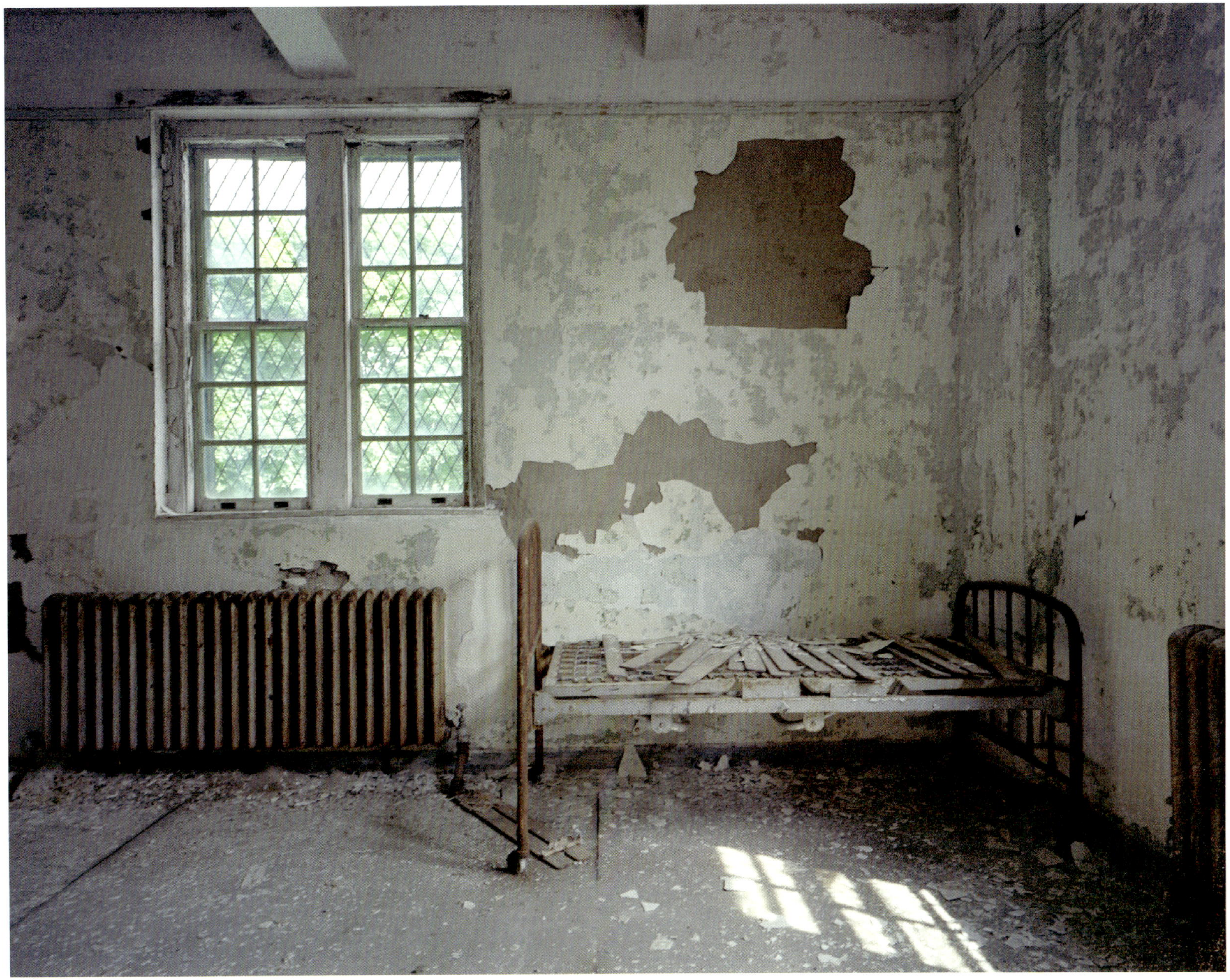

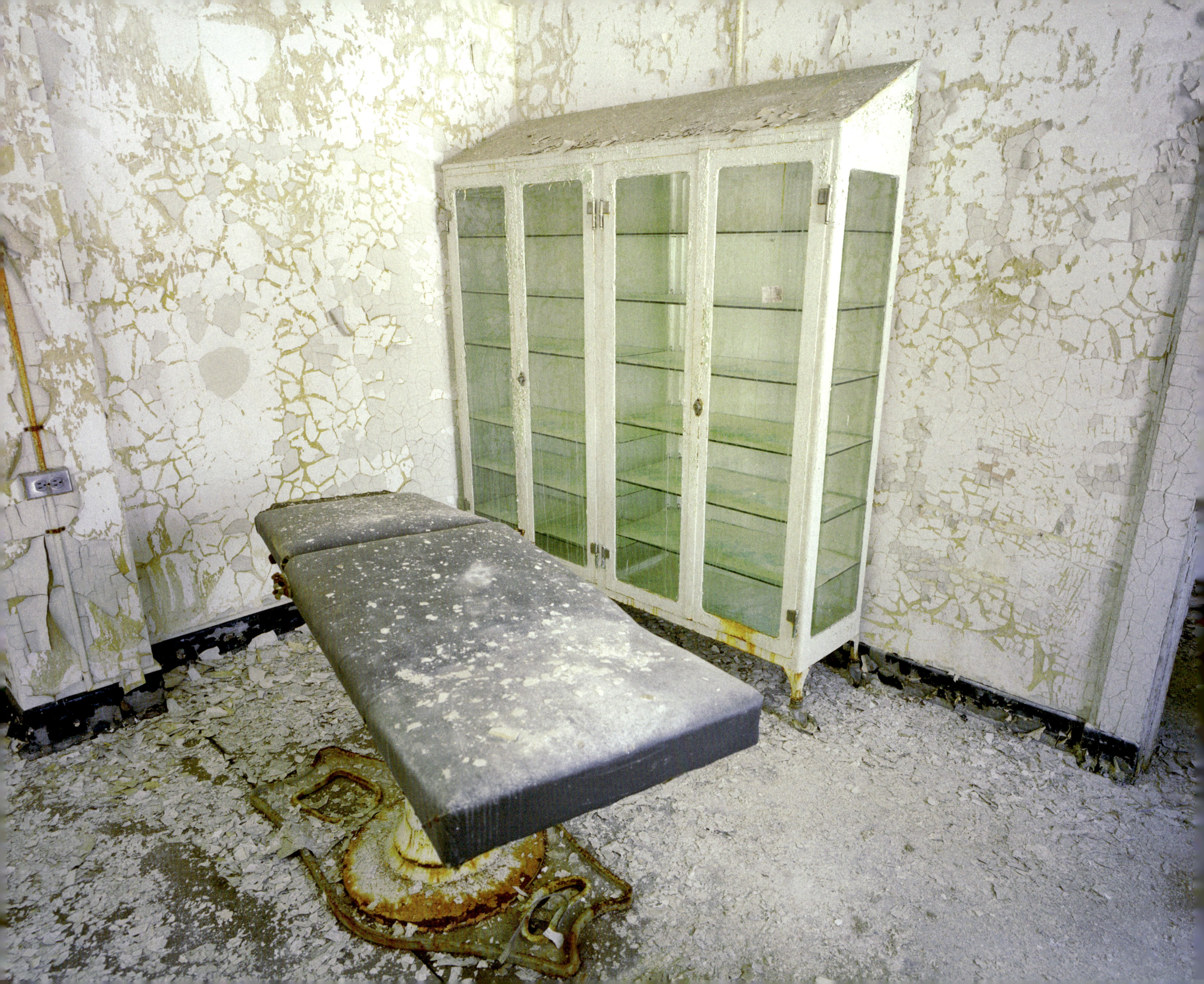

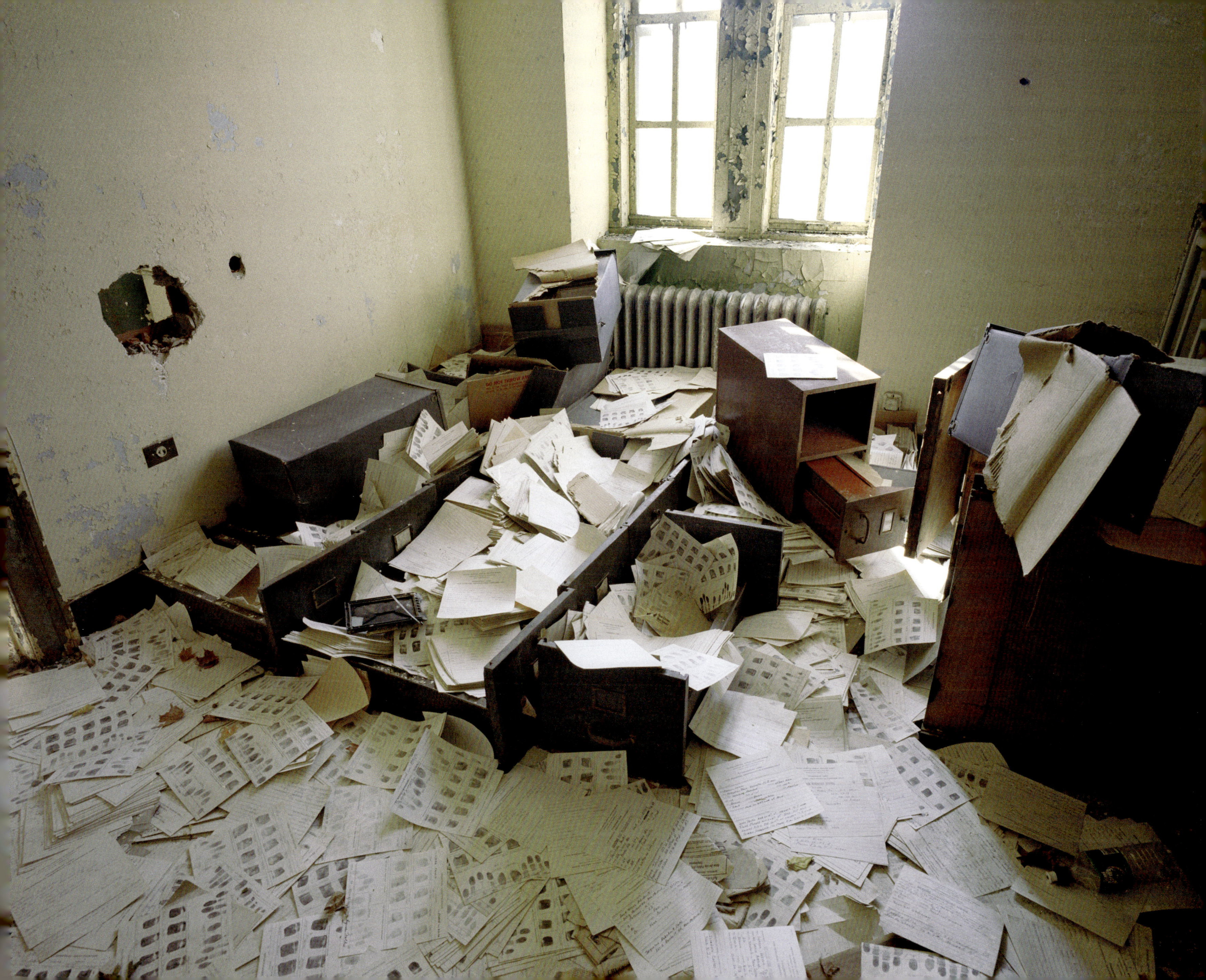

Deary Mary

sixty biggy loneysomey hard months here
since I seed any or alla you

o god please
just a donty ya ever let me suffer
this loneysome without you
way this long no more

If I've ever doney one meany baddy thing
for alla you guys ta be off
on a biggy strikey aginst me
I am hereby apologizin

and I'll be gladdy ta granty you
all all your demands
you ever ever demanden off me

Lovey me
Writey me
$avey me
Lordey god Woody

Woody's letter to his wife Marjorie. August 18, 1956.

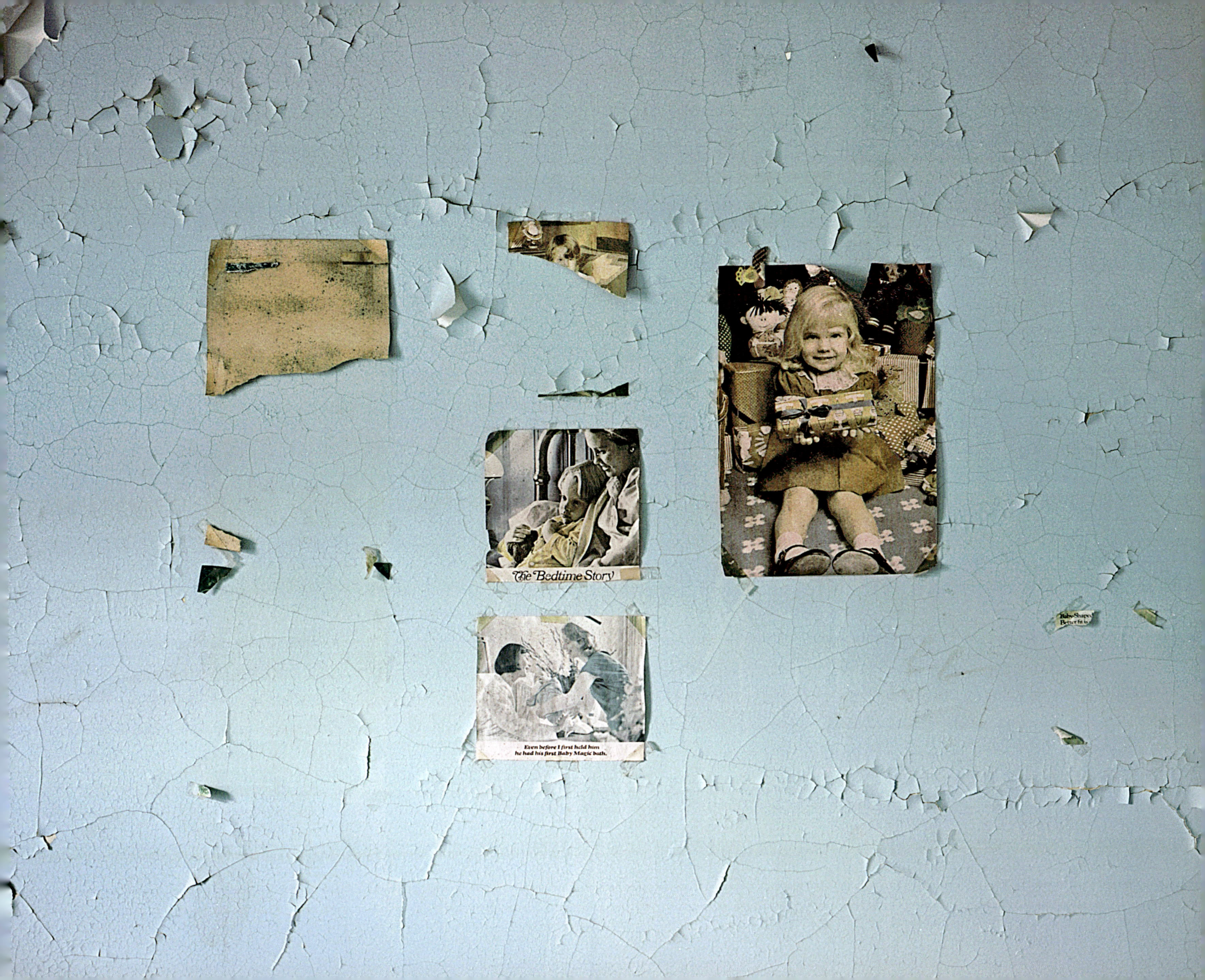
The Bedtime Story
Even before I first held him
he had his first Baby Magic bath.

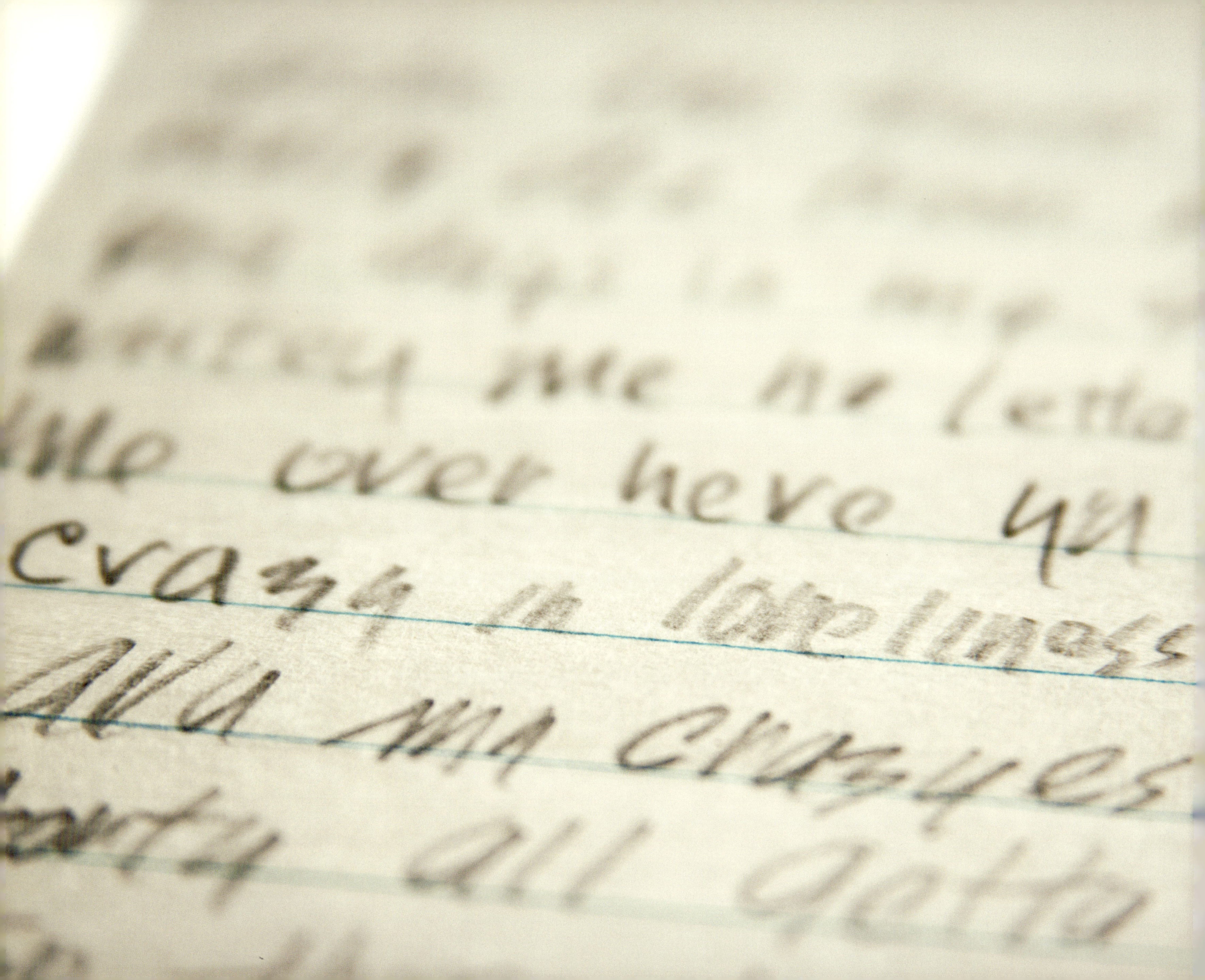
over here
all

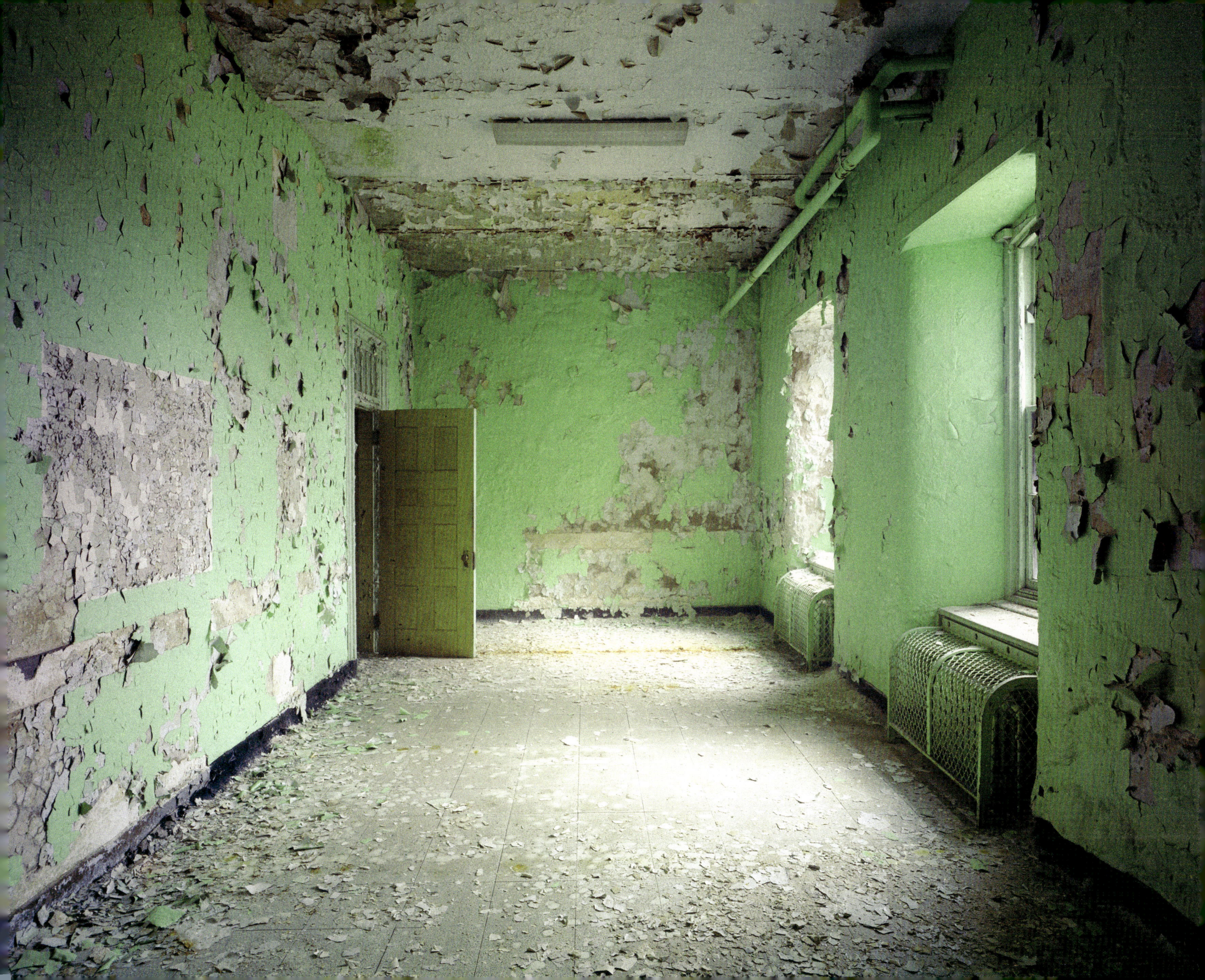

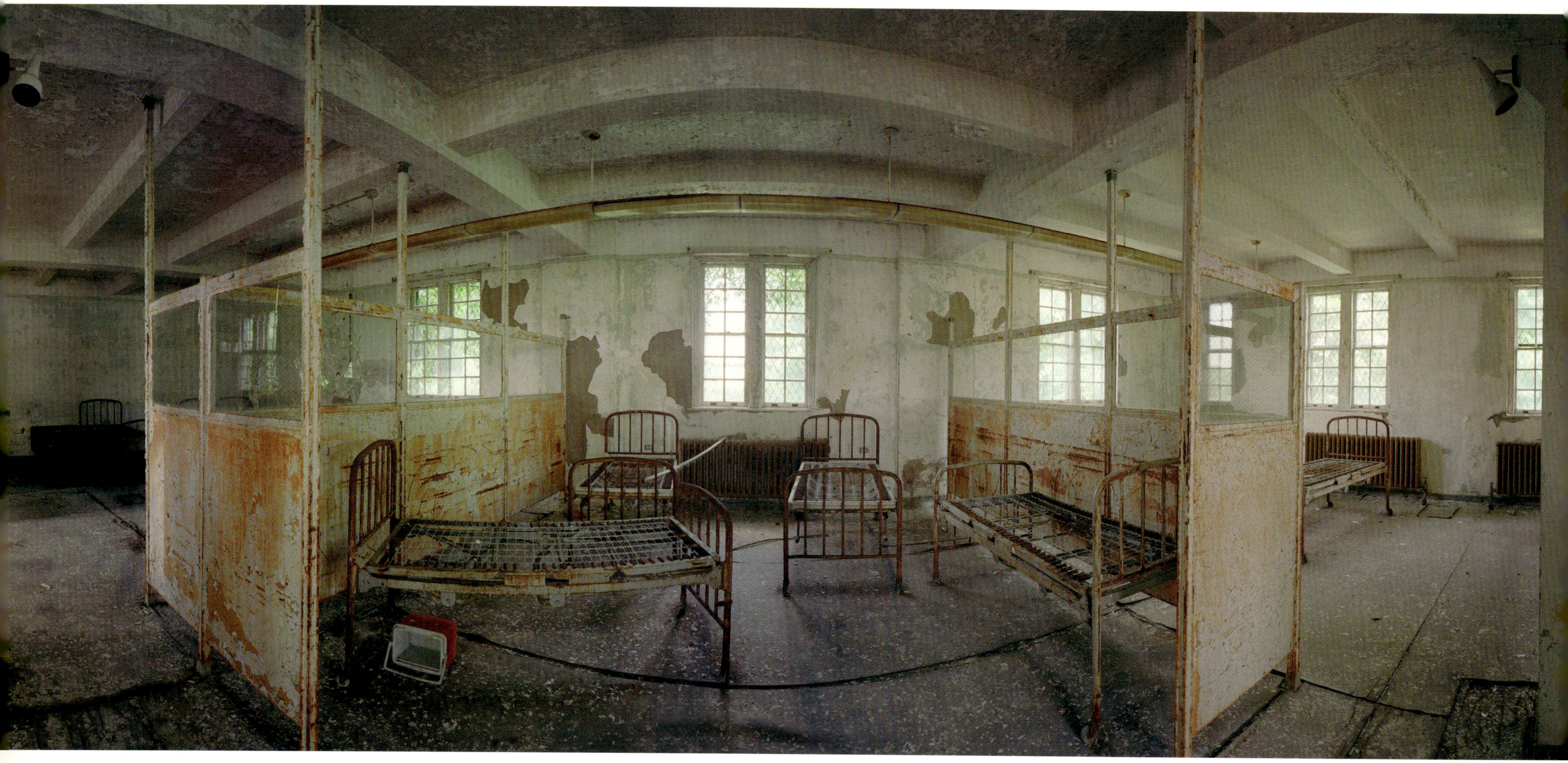

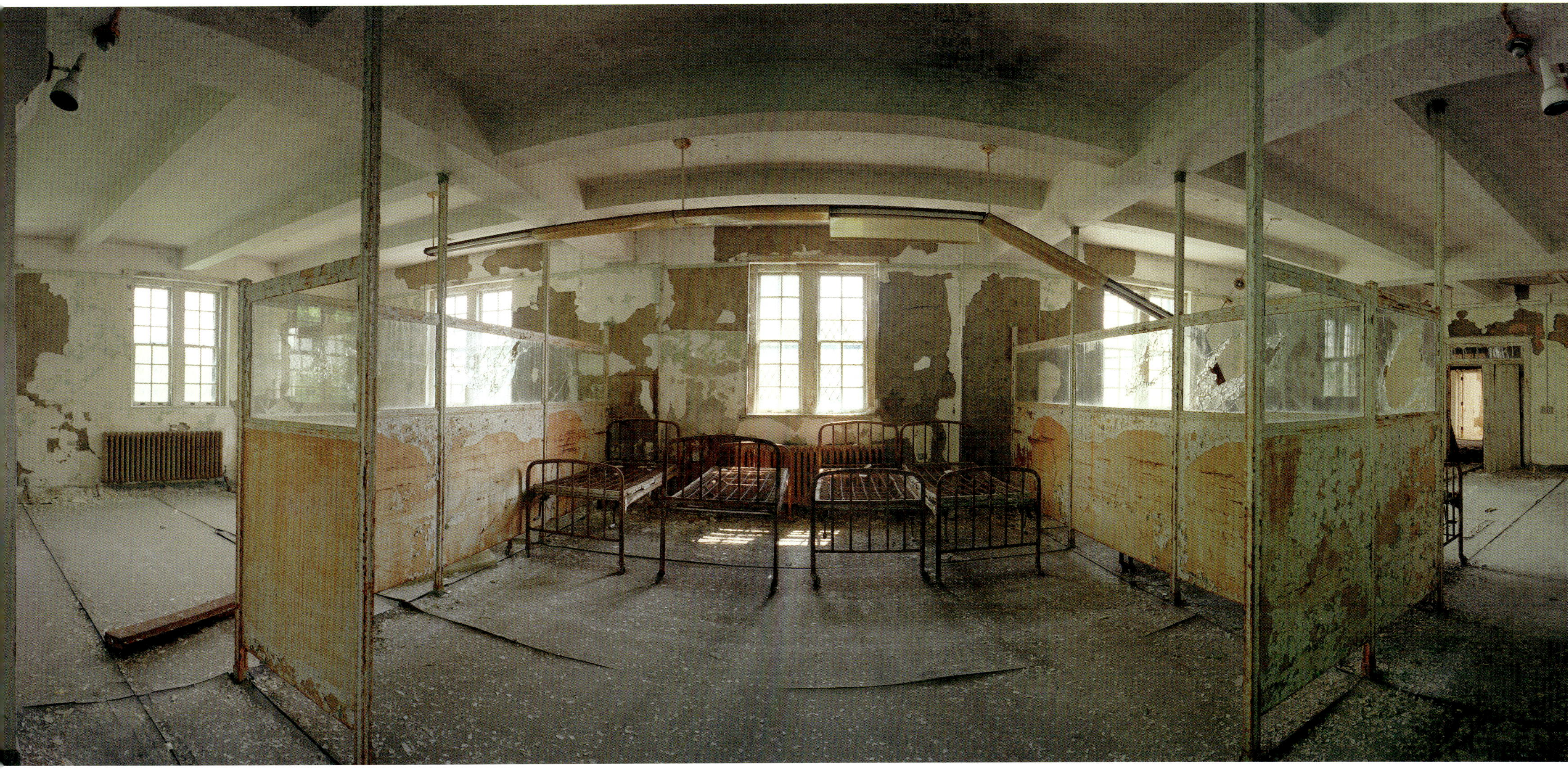

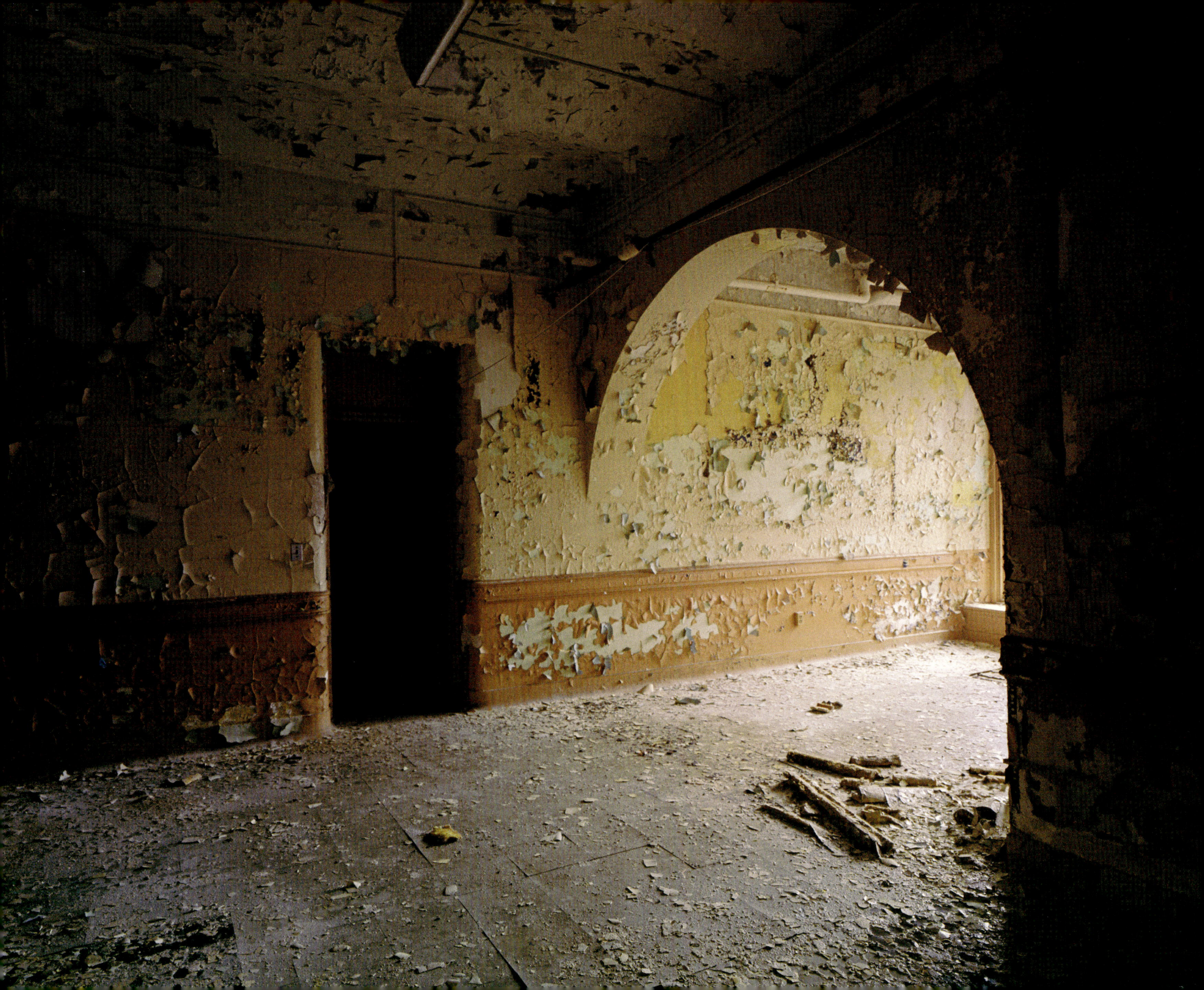

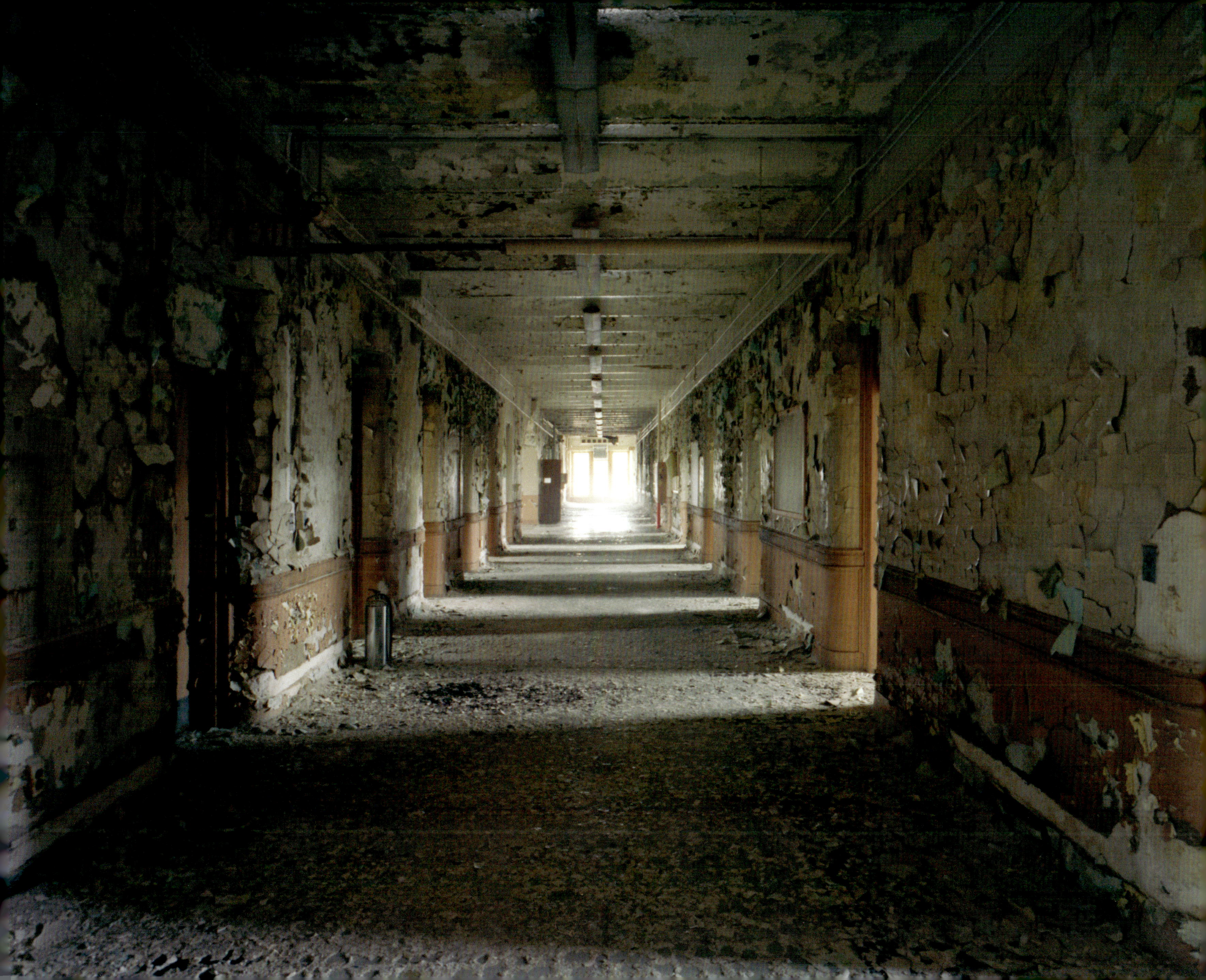

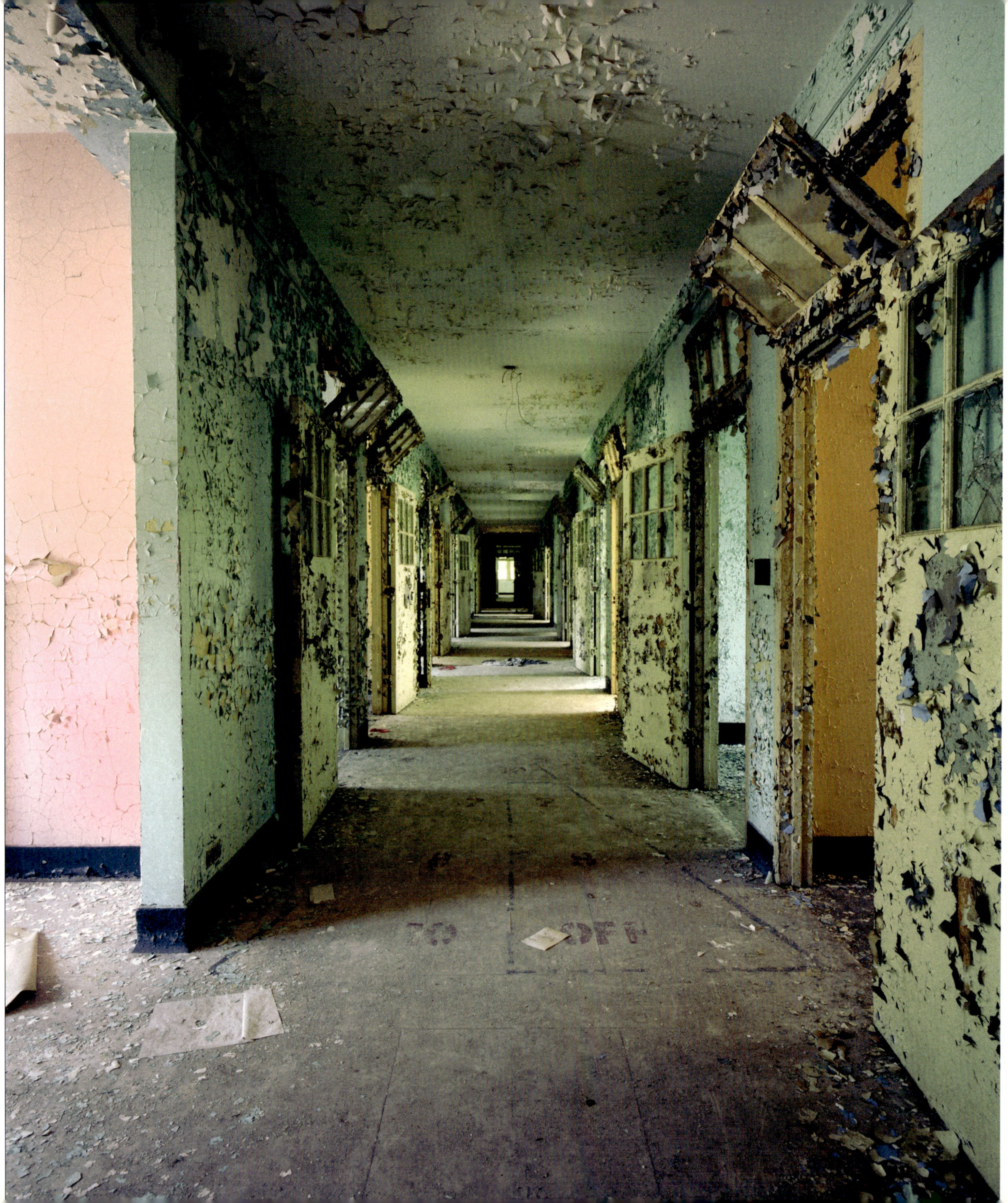

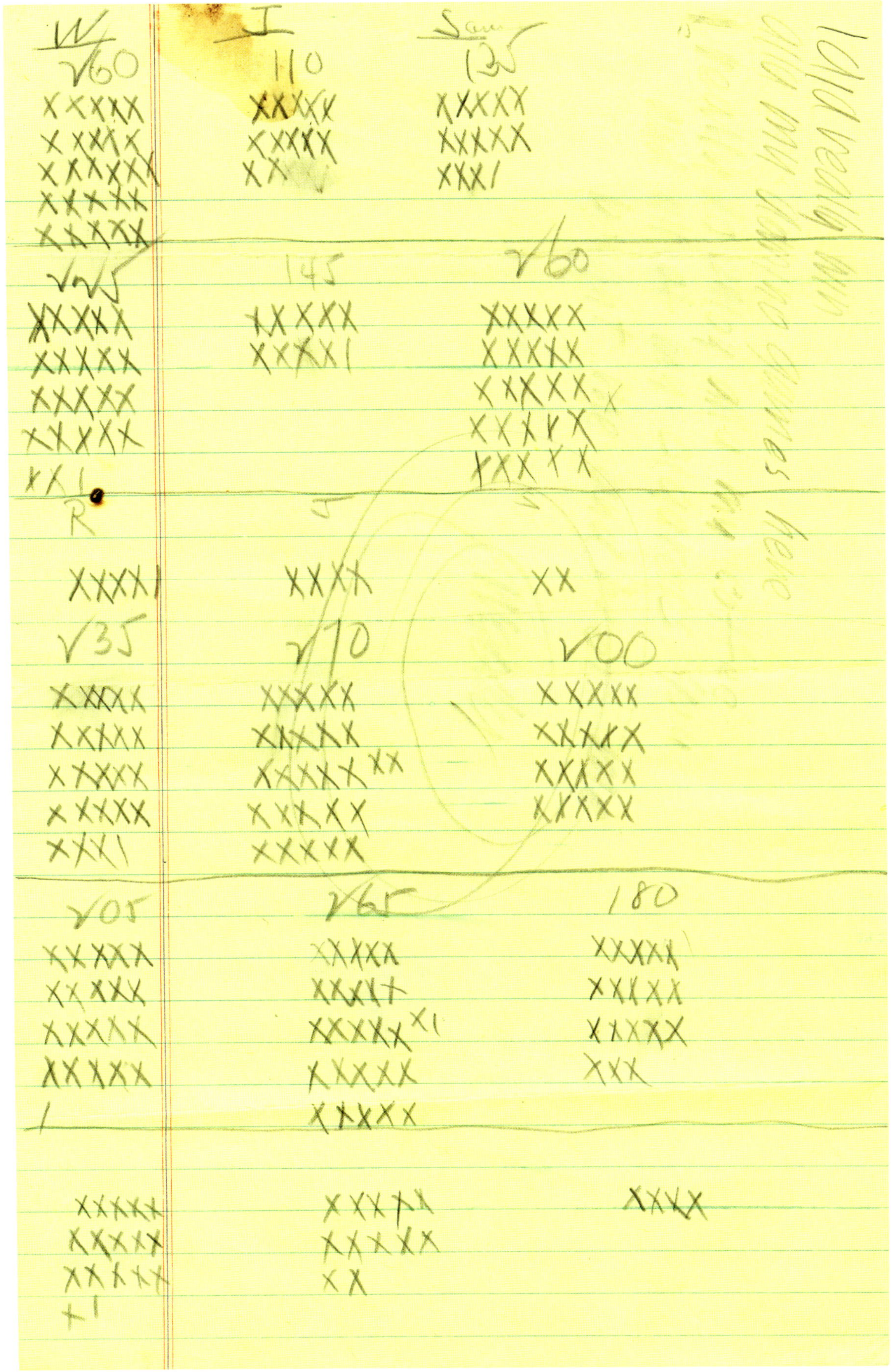

"I did really win alla my domino games here."
Woody. October 22, 1956.

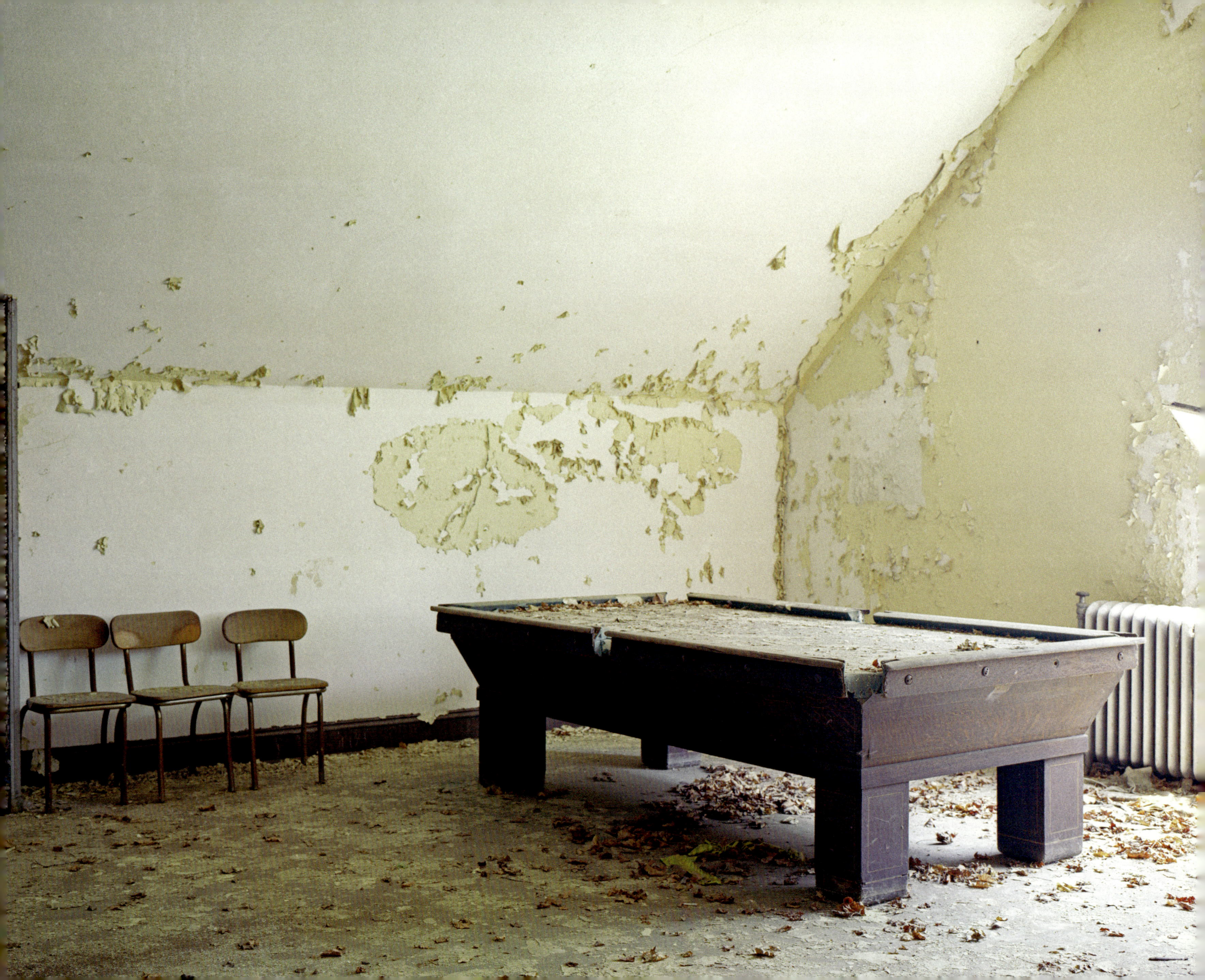

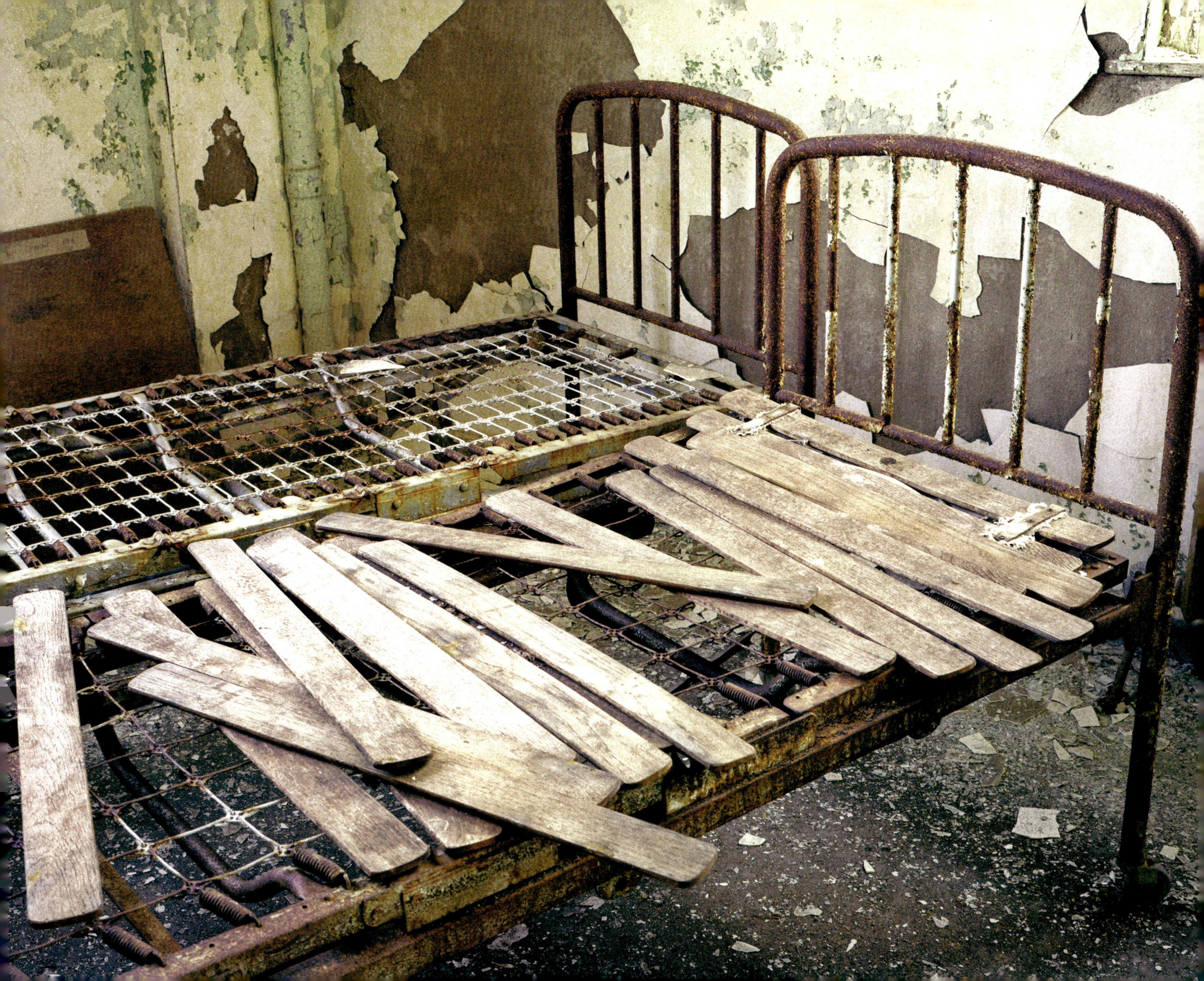

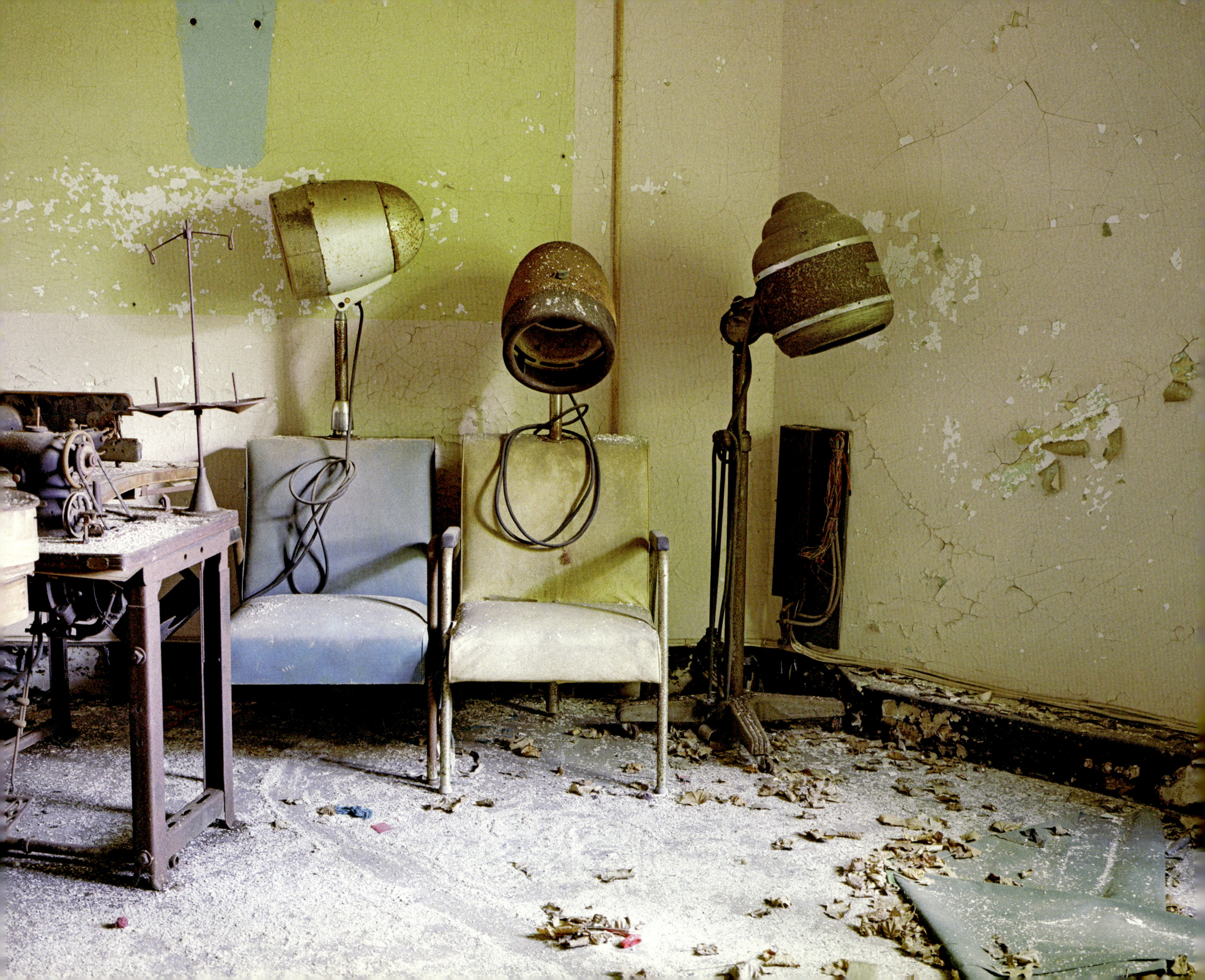

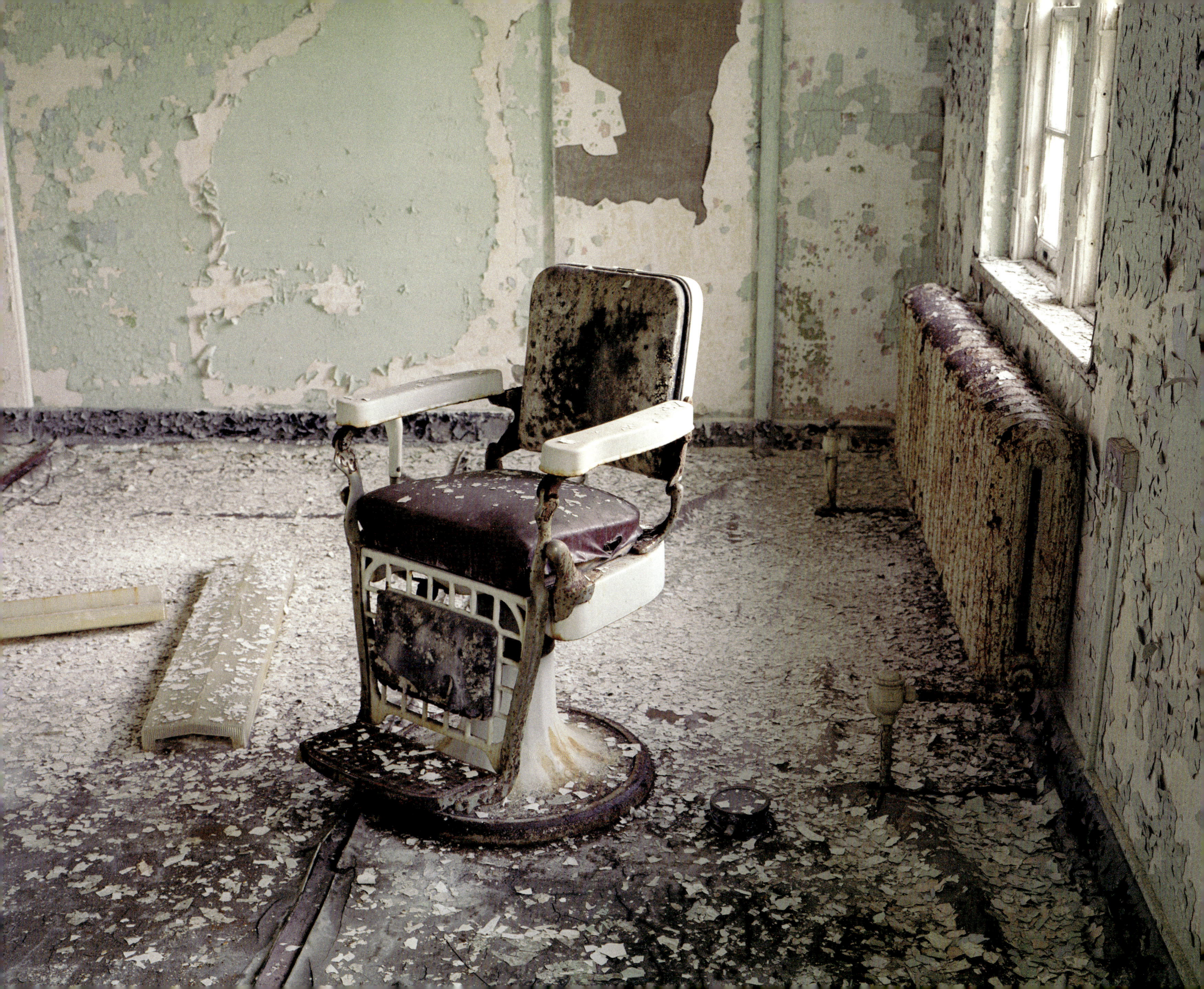

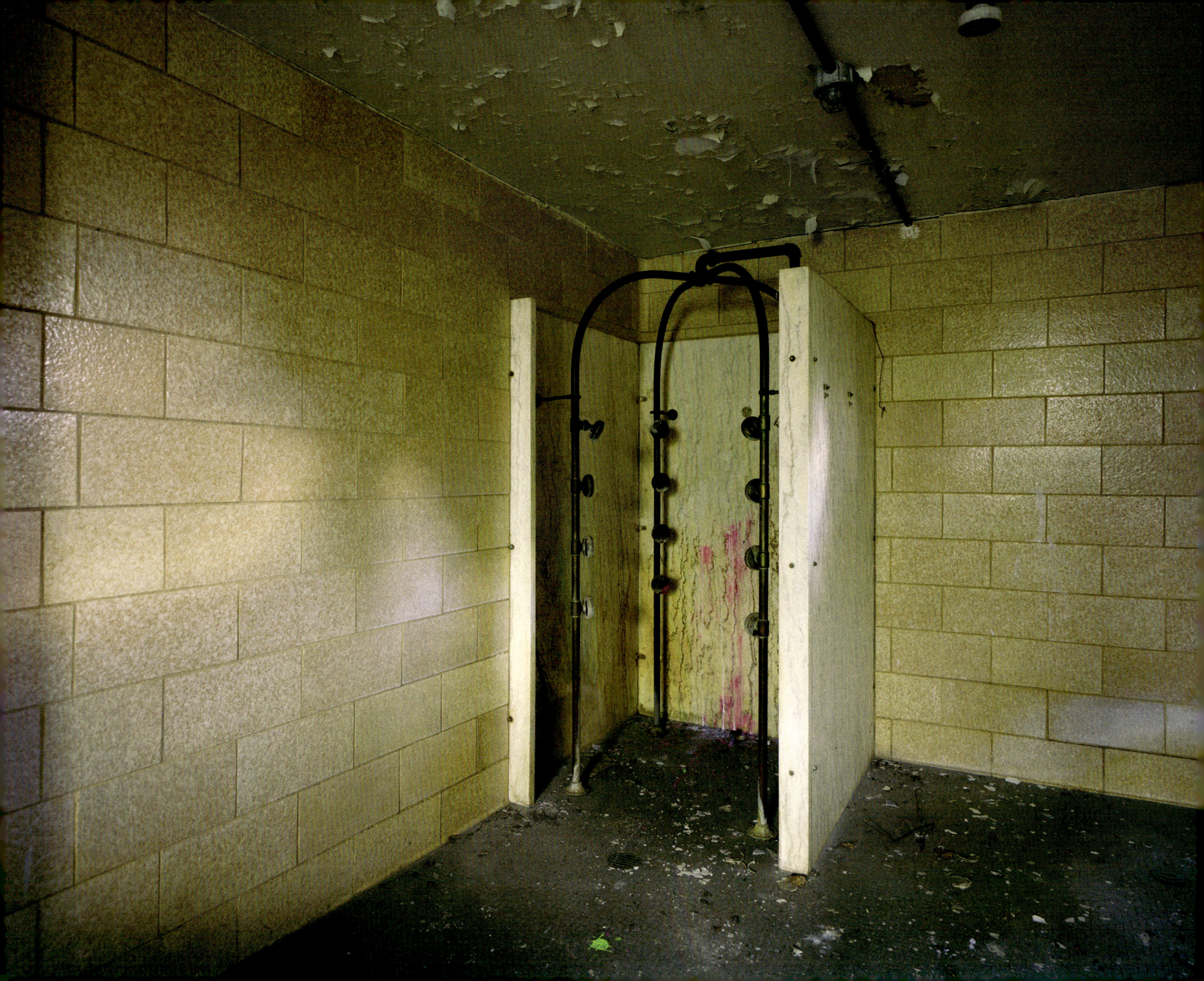

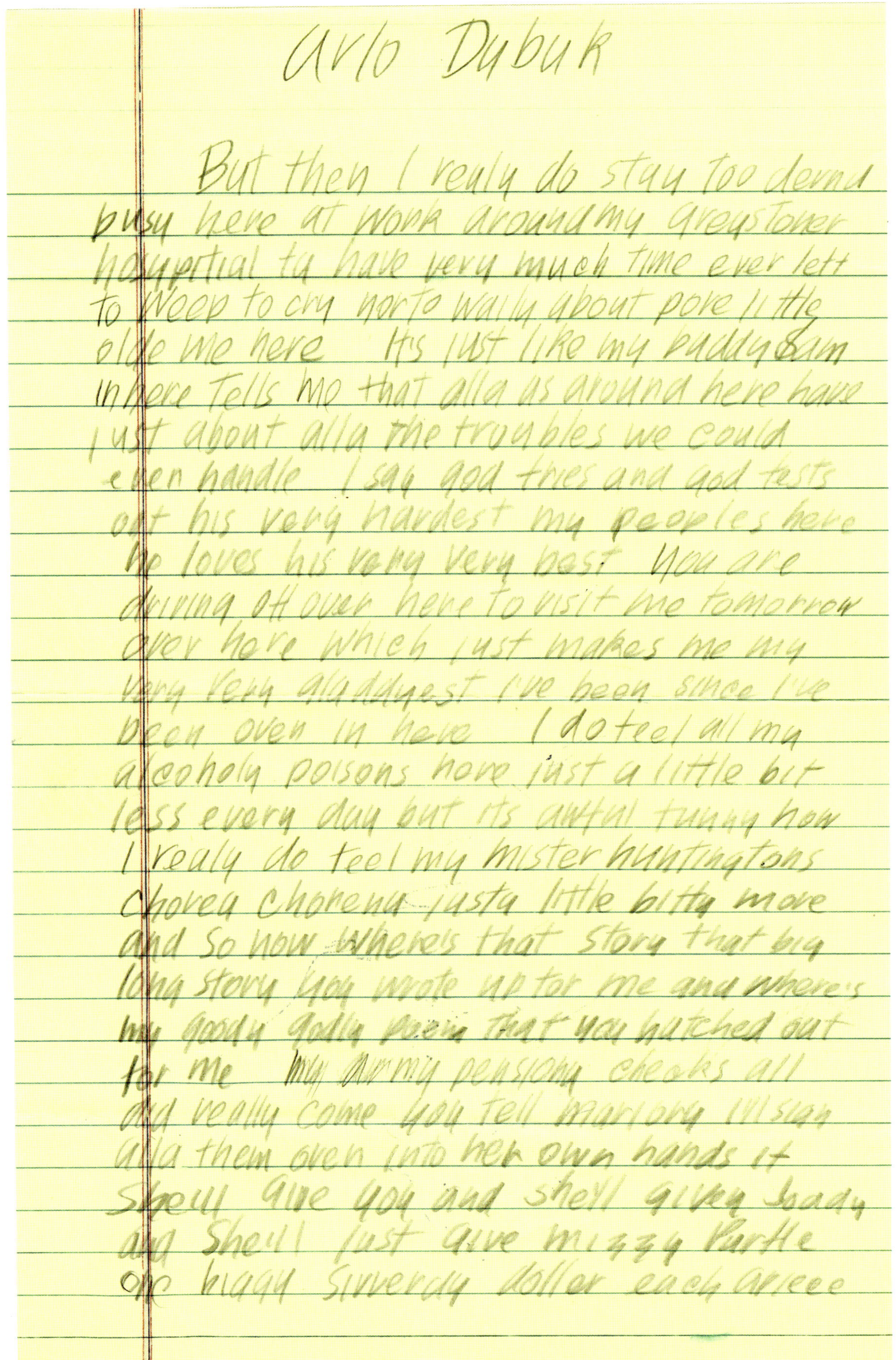

Arlo Dubuk

But then I realy do stay too derned
busy here at work around my Greystoner
hosprtial ta have very much time ever left
to weep to cry nor to wally about pore little
olde me here. It's just like my buddy Sam
in here tells me that alla us around here have
just about alla the troubles we could
even handle. I say God tries and God tests
out his very hardest my peoples here
he loves his very very best. You are
driving off over here to visit me tomorrow
over here which just makes me my
very very gladdyest I've been since I've
been oven in here. I do feel all my
alcoholy poisons hove just a little bit
less every day but its awful funny how
I realy do feel my mister huntingtons
Chorey Chorena justa little bitty more
And so now where's that story that big
long story you wrote up for me and where's
my goody godly poem that you hatched out
for me. My army pensiony checks all
did really come you tell Marjory Mason
alla them oven into her own hands it
She'll give you and she'll give Joady
and She'll just give Mizzy Purtle
one biggy silverdy dollar each apiece

Woody's letter to his son Arlo. 1956.

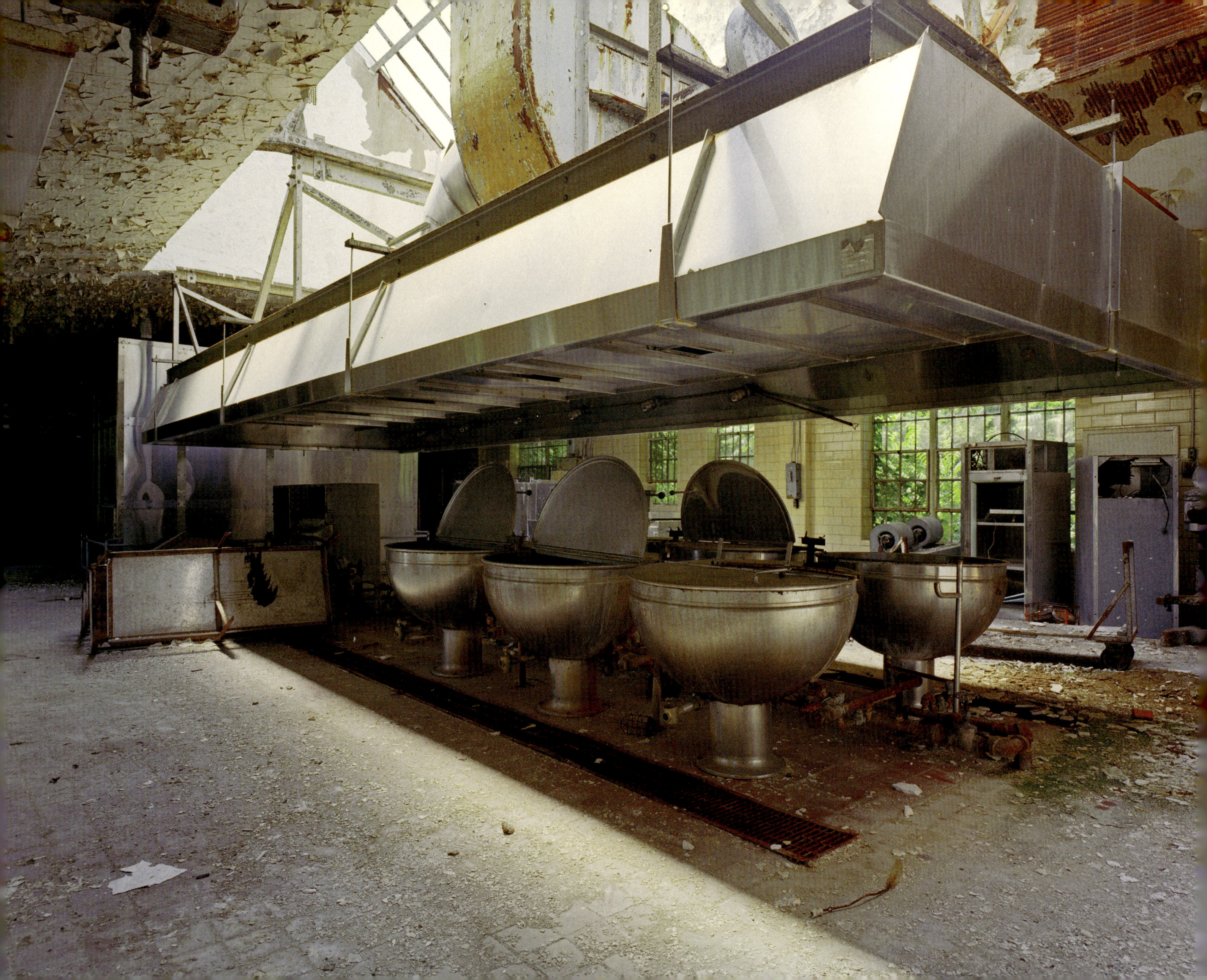

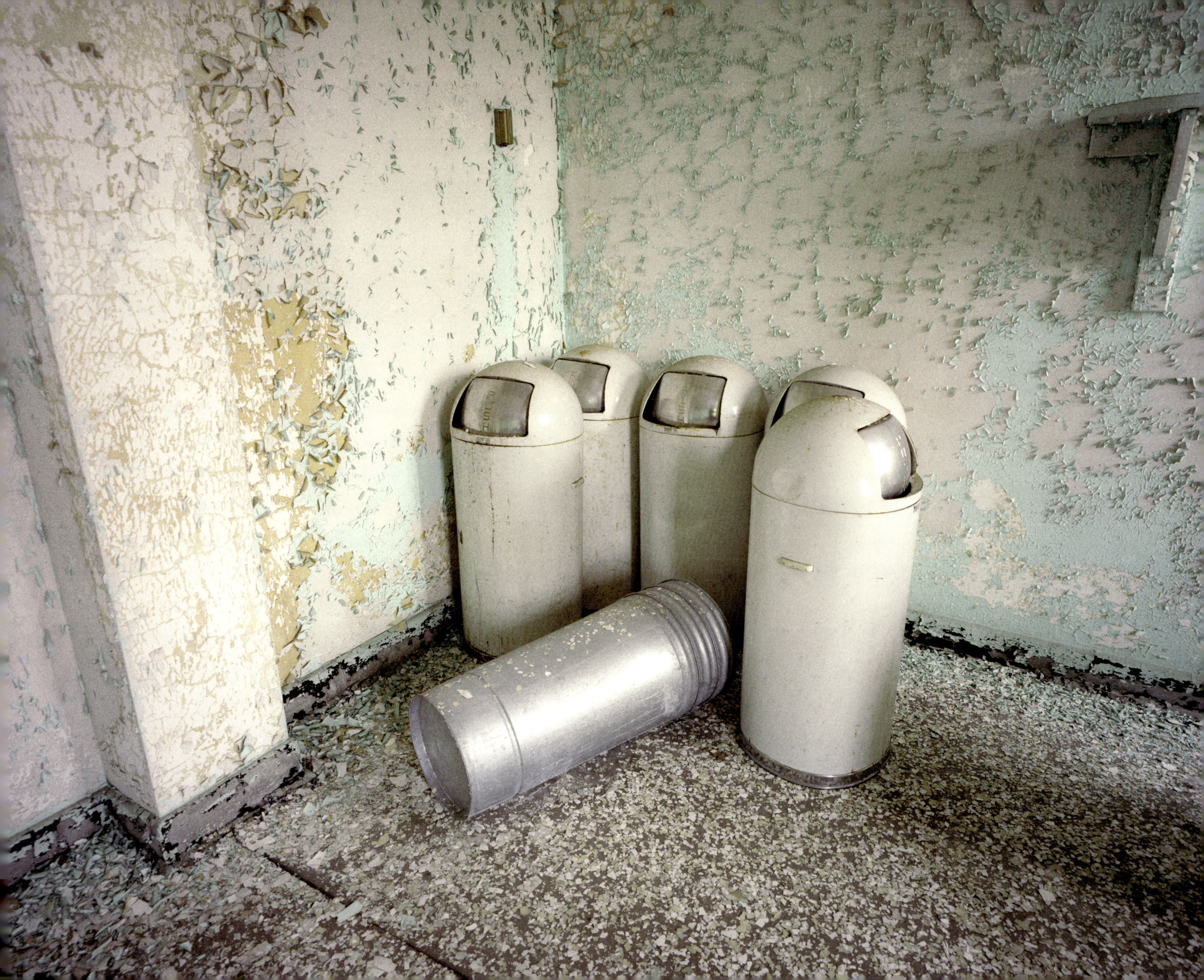

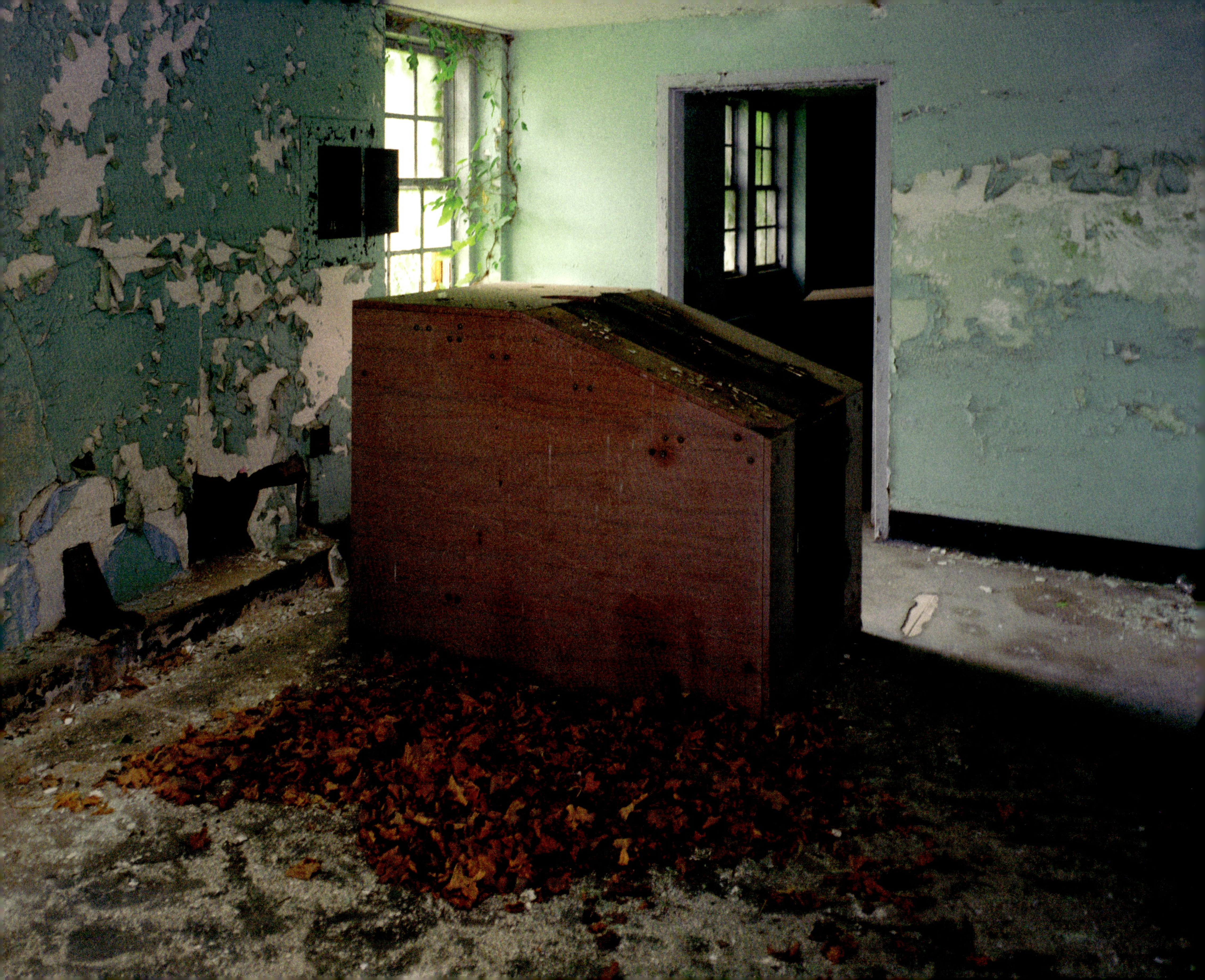

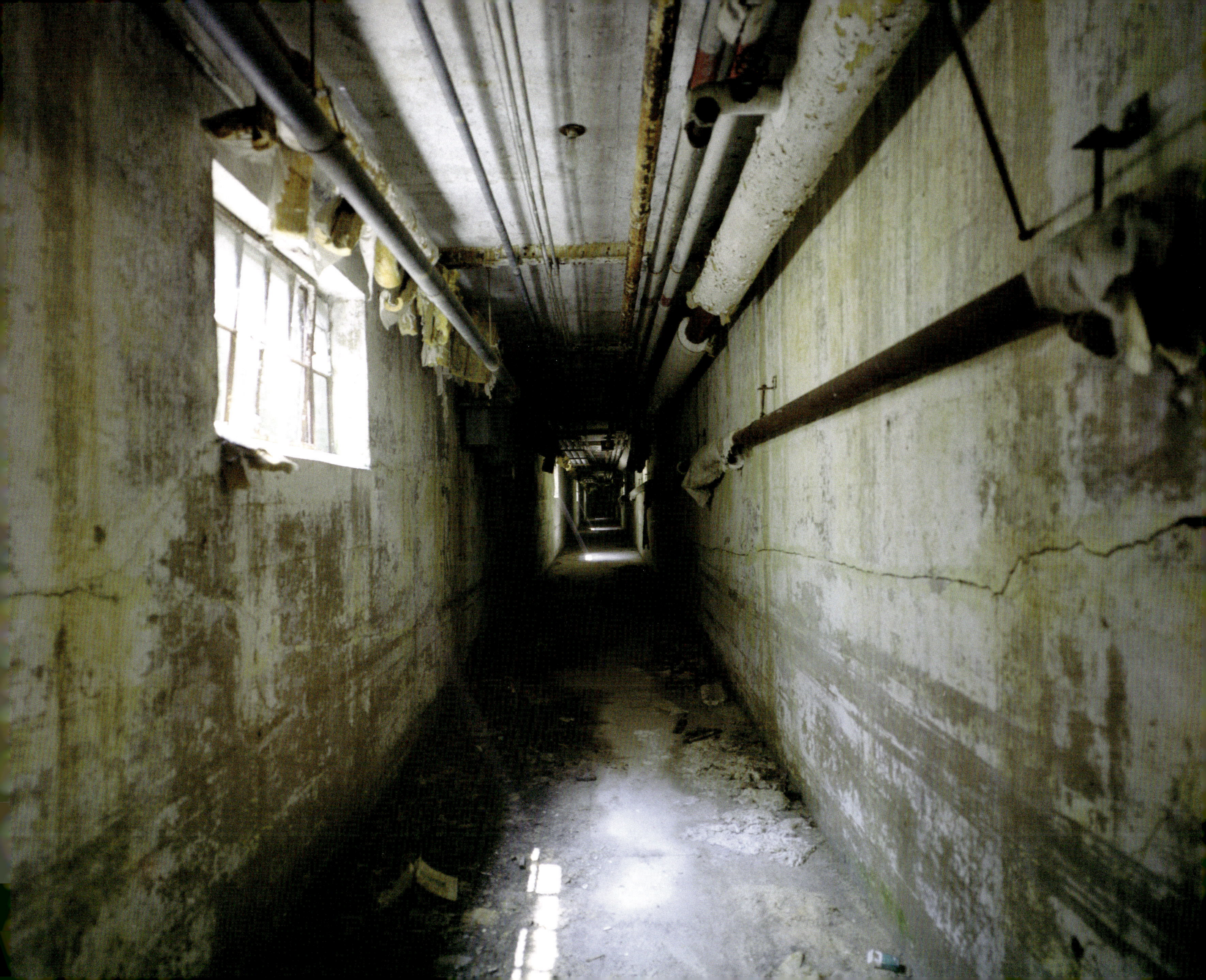

Marjy

But What makes every man along here
in my wardy forty
o yes my lordy
what makes my old whole Wardy torty here
run tight and fly so fast
tu grabby just one little puff here
off my cegaretty
tag tag draggy drag drag

and marjy telly me pleasy
am I really gettin ta be a fiend
for thoryzene

Me daddy Woody

Woody's letter to his wife, Marjorie. October 4, 1956

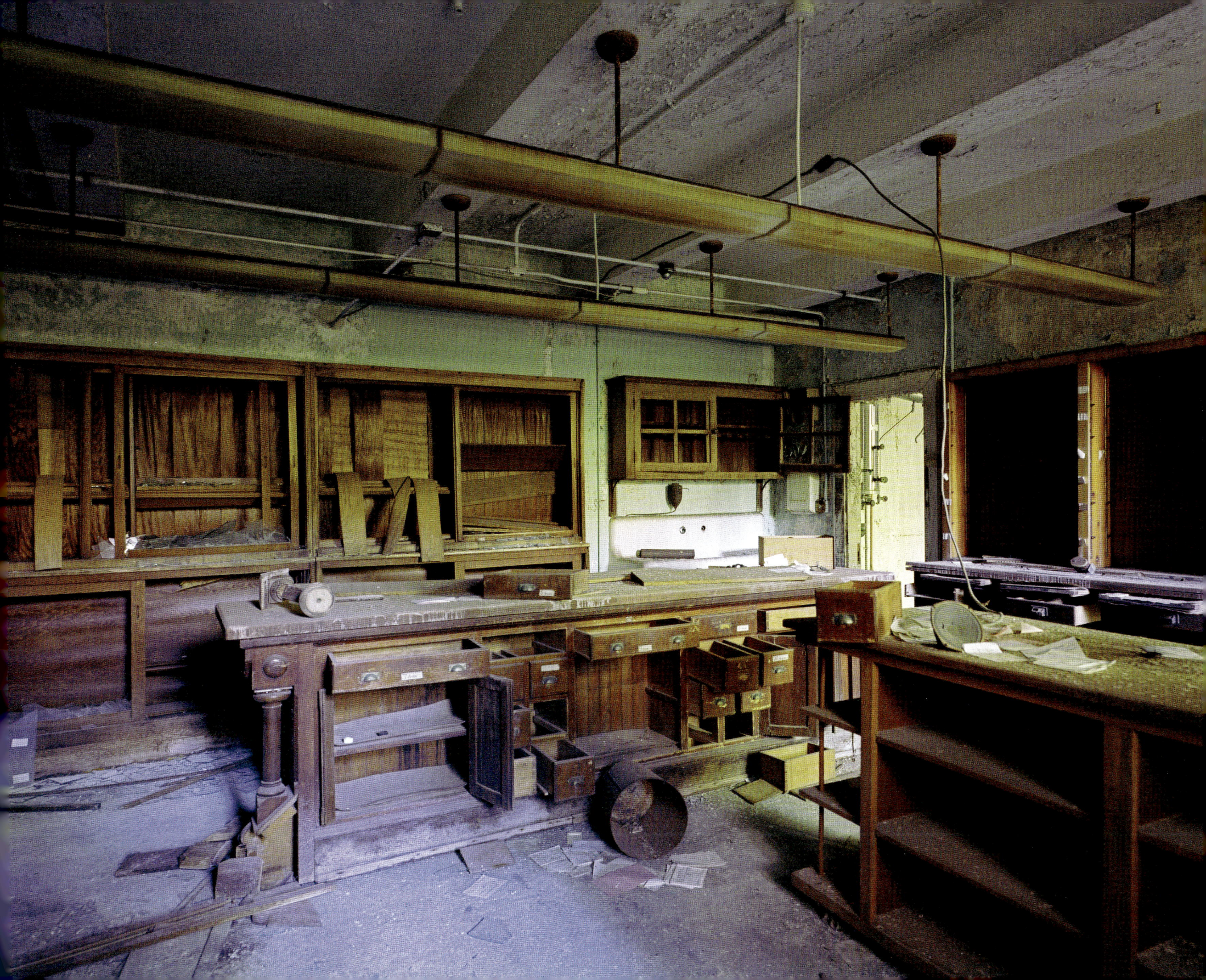

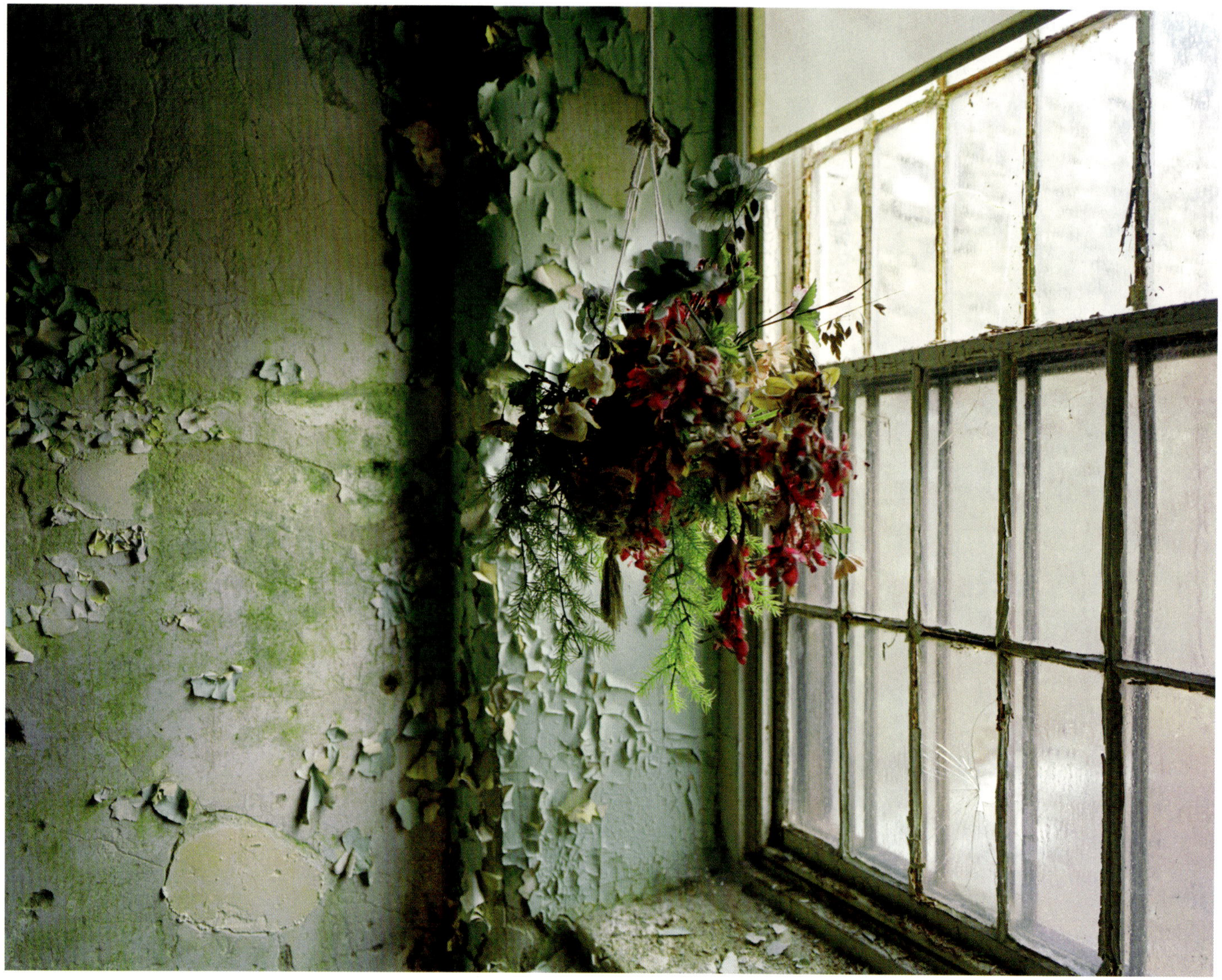

Arlo Bee

Woody Guthrie ☆

Your picturdy card gave me my
best goody reason tu go on alvin I guess
we put fresh watery pottyd flowers all up
and down my ward here to make me
smella huley lots nicer Write me more
pray for me ameny aginy
Your dadey Arlo
tell me about teenys family

Woody's letter to his son, Arlo. 1956.

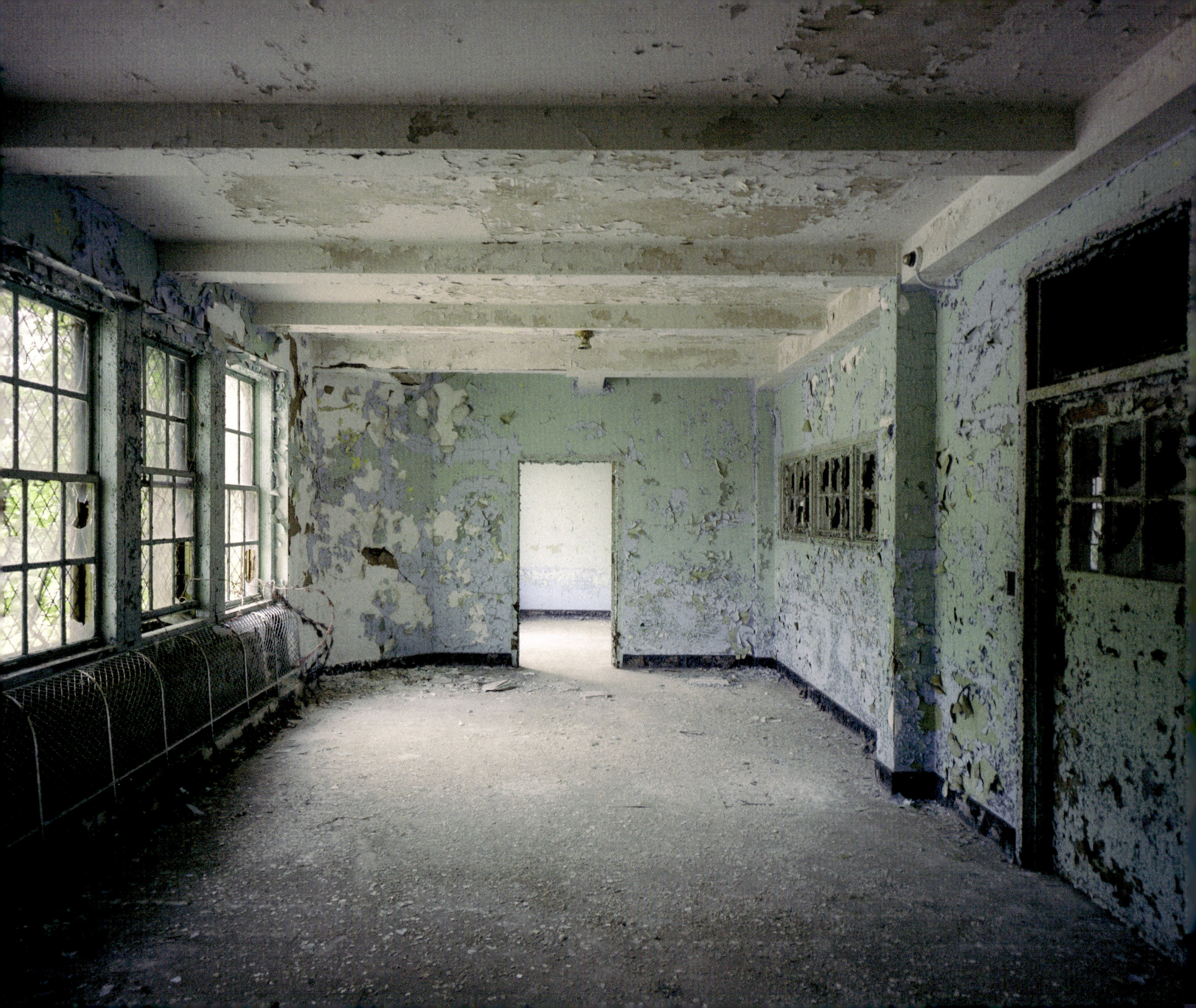

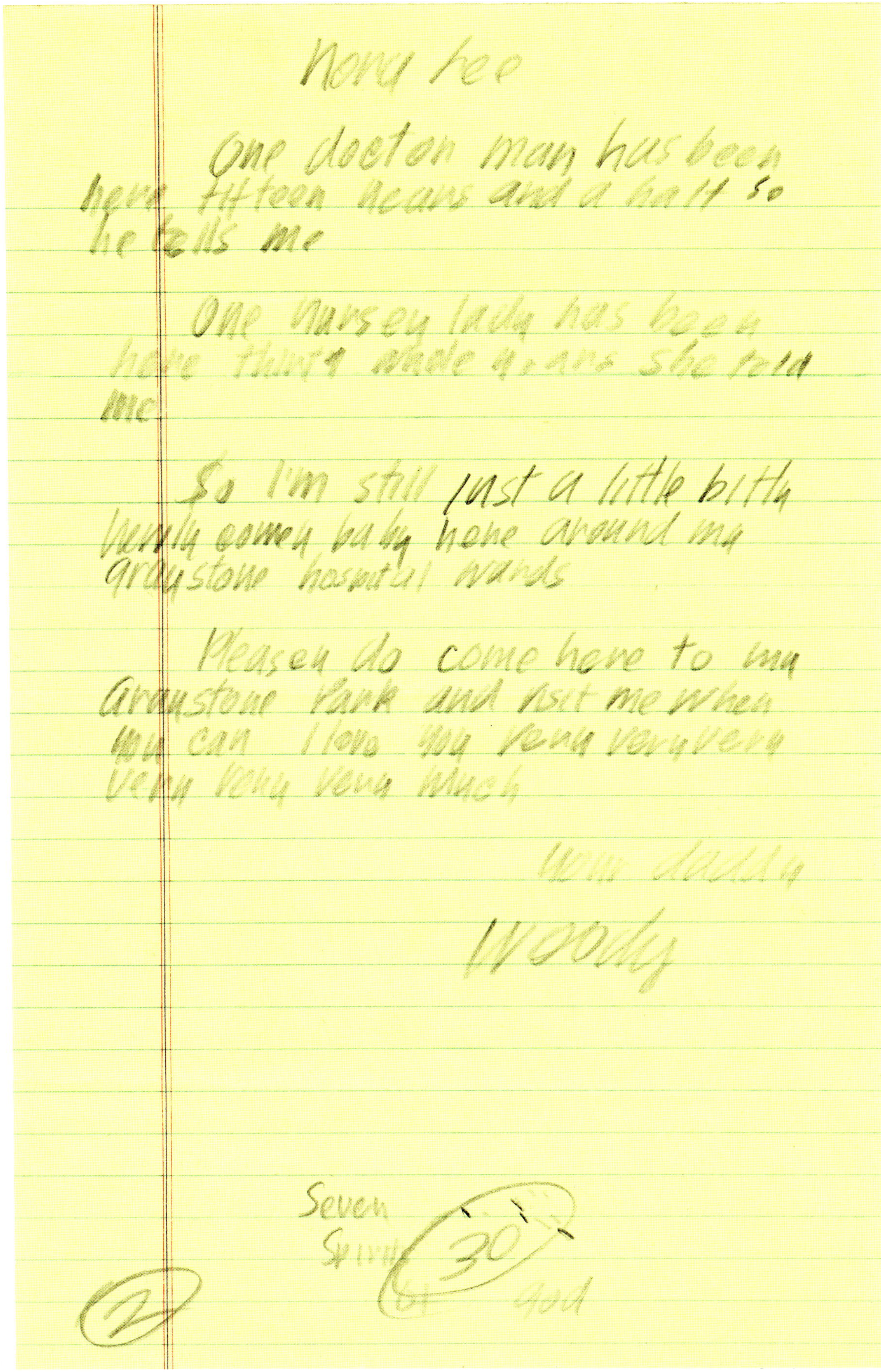

Nora Lee

One doctor man has been here fifteen years and a half so he tells me

One nursey lady has been here thirty whole years she told me

So I'm still just a little bitty teeny weeny baby here around my graystone hospital wards

Pleasey do come here to my Graystone Park and visit me when you can I love you very very very very very very much

Your daddy

Woody

Seven
Seven
30
God

2

Woody's letter to his daughter, Nora Lee. 1956.

I don't remember if it was the first or the second, but we took a car, drove out there, this huge building looked like from the 1880s, and we were then told it was an insane asylum and Woody was in this place. We went in to see Woody, and he was in less–than–good condition. But the interesting part of it is he didn't say, "Get me out of here." We would talk to the attendants or the doctors and try to tell them who he was or what he did. They were skeptical about it. At times he would tell me he wanted a guitar, and the next visit I would bring out a guitar. One visit, he wanted a record player, and I'd bring one out. And as I would come out, I'd have to take stuff back because he couldn't handle it. He couldn't handle the guitar, and even the record machine was a problem for him.–*Harold Leventhal*

Harold Leventhal, Woody, and Lou Gordon. 1960.

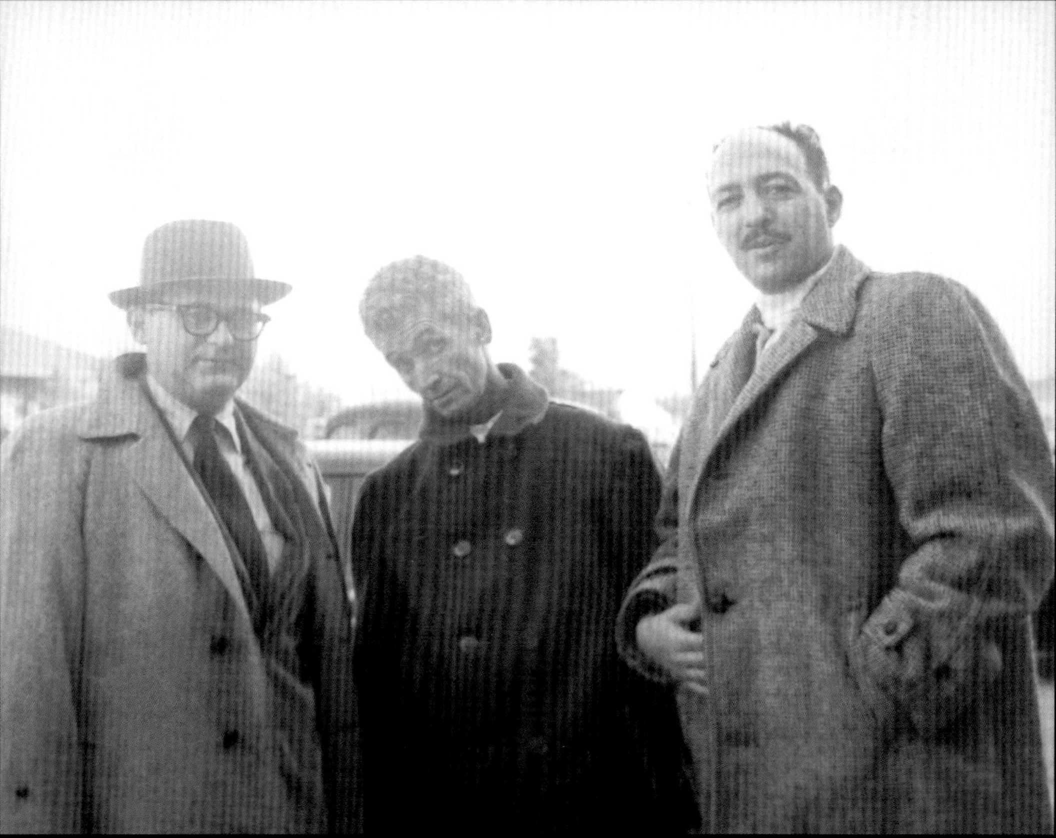

And then, within a short time he's in this ward–they didn't know where to put him–where he's with other people who they consider, like him, to be mentally deranged. And so that's whom he's talking to, who he's hanging out with everyday. No one knows who he is. But then one day another patient comes over and says, "I know who you are. You're Woody Guthrie, the famous singer." He says, "Yes, I am." The guy says, "I loved your book, "Bound for Glory." "You read my book?" "No, I ate your book." I mean, moments like that are probably the few highlights of his time there, you know.–*Arlo Guthrie*

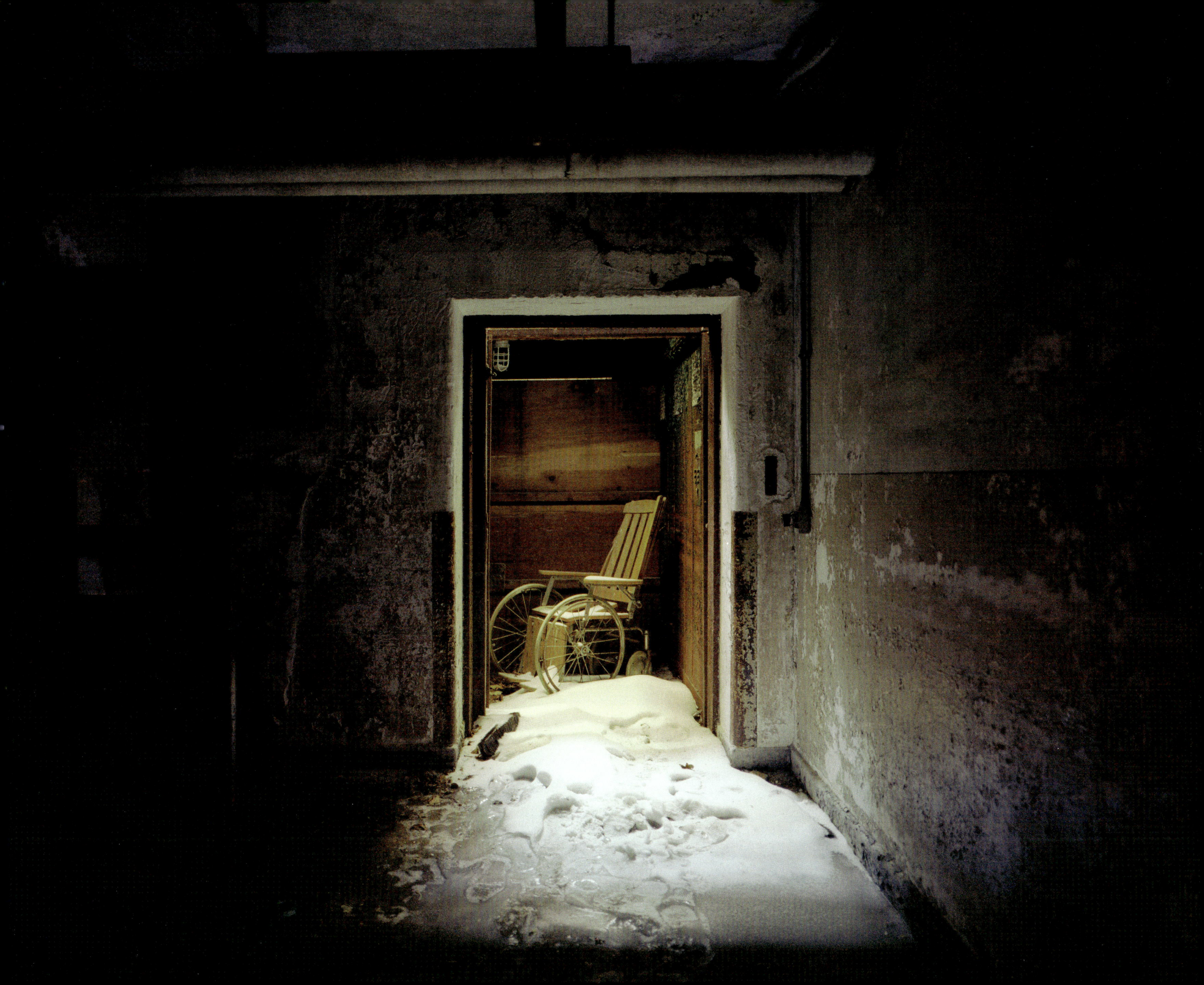

He took care of the people that were there, Woody did. There were just a lot of people there, and sometimes he'd play guitar for them, and sometimes the harmonica, and he'd walk outside, he liked to go out and sit in the sun, and all things like that.–*Sidsel Gleason*

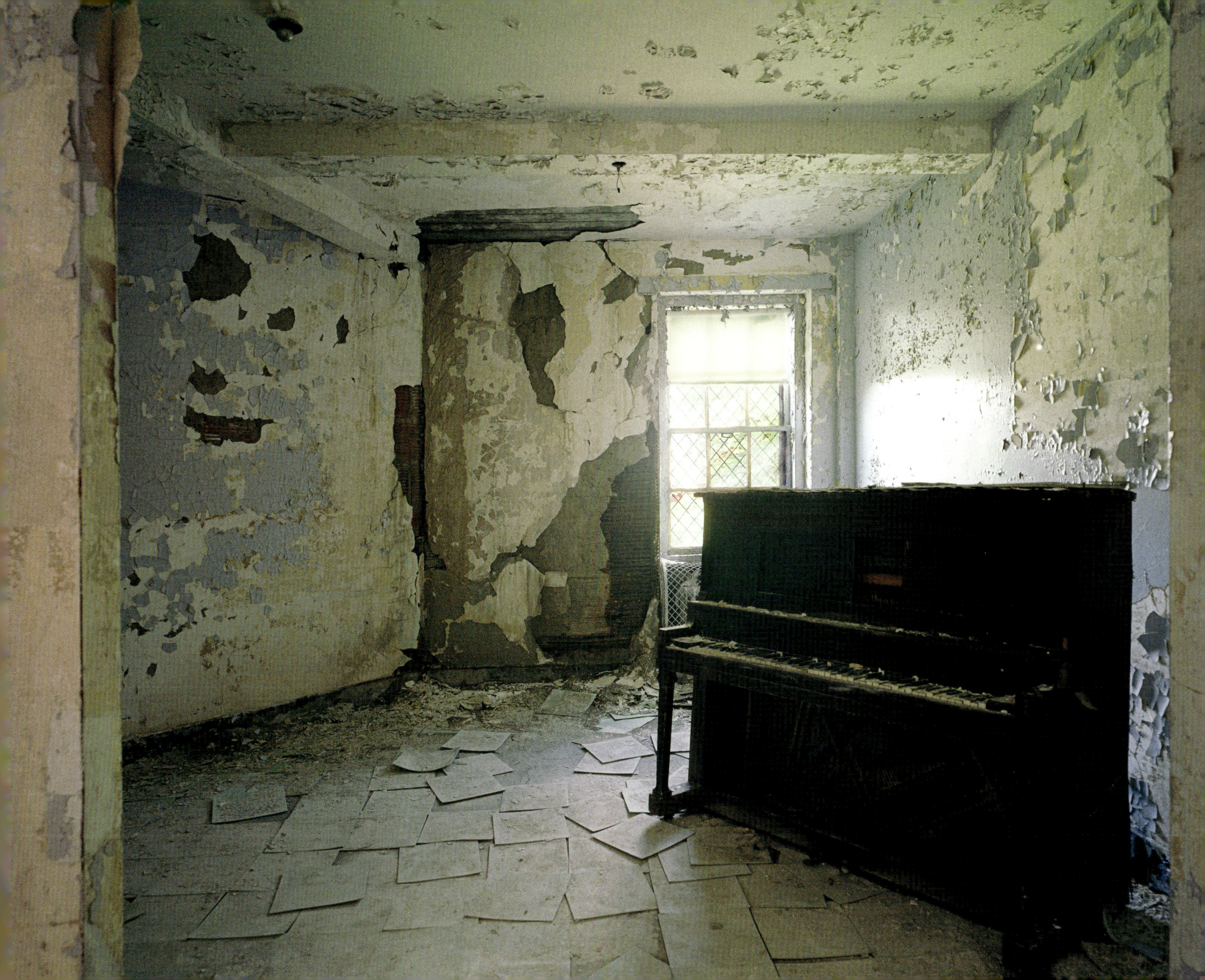

I did walk along and I do stand up here in my window on my good wardy forty lordy and I do look out down here and I see my same 80 crazy guys acting out every one of my antics I did write you all about in my play I named my forsakern bible.*–Woody's letter to his daughter Nora Lee, October 22, 1956*

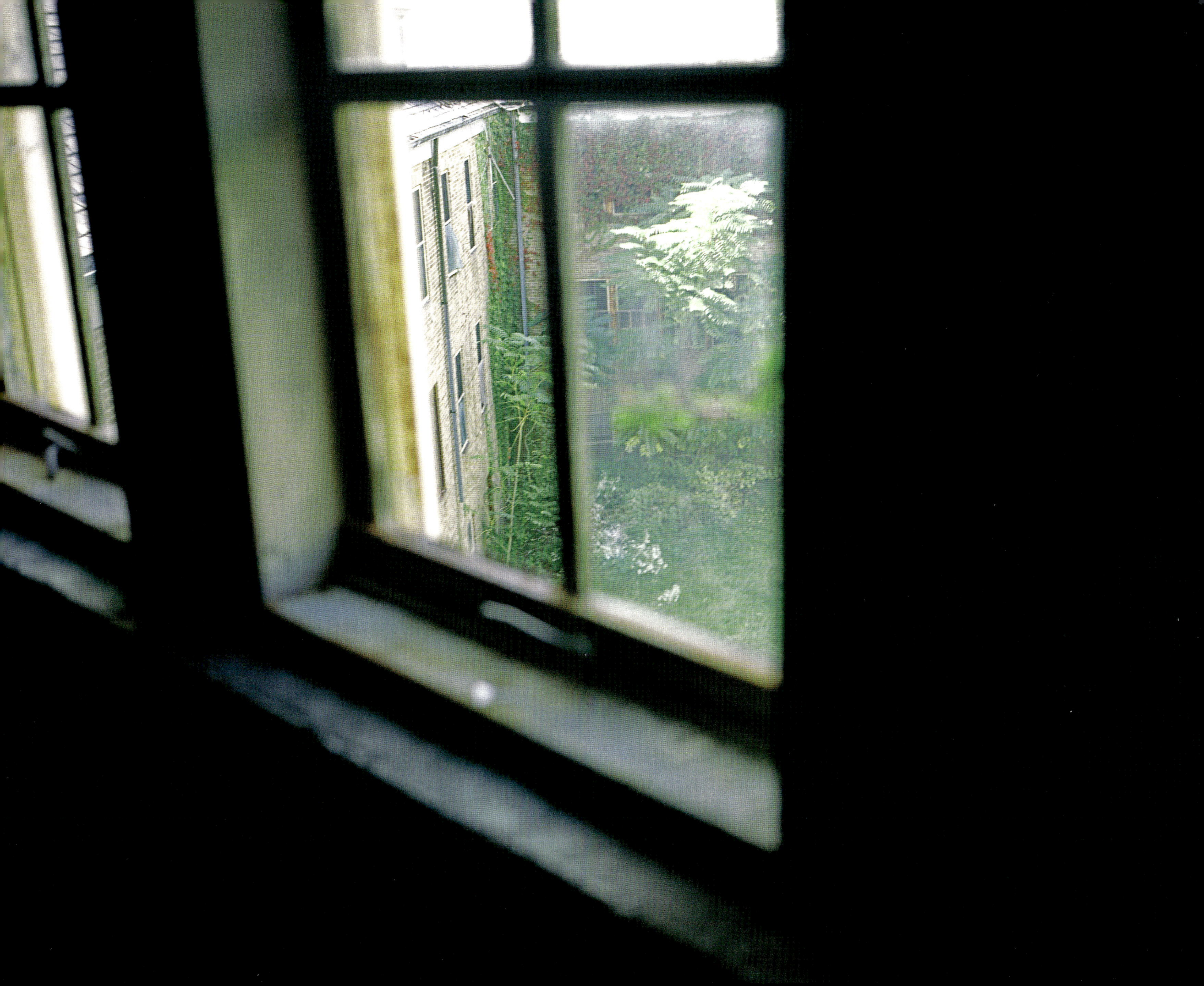

Woody:

It sure beats other kinds of factory work and other kindsa jobs 'cause I savin', salvagin' all good human souls, spirits and bodies. It makes Ward 40 the very best ship I ever did ride on. And I did ride on boats through four invasions—North Aferkee, Sicily, D-Day and through V-bomber raids over London.

Old Shaker Man:

But this is a bigger battle here in old ward 40.

Woody:

Just a damn site bigger. Lots better fight goin' on around my old ward here. My big fight against ever' kind of disease, every kind of damn sickyness I seeta be botherin' human kind. All the other big boats cracked you to pieces and dumped you down here. My old Ward 40 takes all these broken up lots pieces of folks and I try my derndnest to stitcher and sew 'em all back together. Oh, God, I try to piece together all your broken pieces so once more you're all better'd up and fixend up all better. . .

Jerry:

Say there Woody, just how does your mother's chorea hit you?

Woody:

Hit my mother Nora Belle when she was about 40. Made her just go into such violent fits and such violent kinds of spasms that, well, she just wreckd and she just wracked every single house we did live in. My cardiographer over yonder in Brooklyn just told me my mother's chorea just sorta passled on to me here. That's about all I really do know about this dang'd fooly stuff.

It just hit me when I was about 40 years old and my muscles all, all, they do just sorta twitchy and just sorta go jumpin' around anywheres that they dang well please, without me ever havin' myself one single damny little word to say about it. Alla my joints here, just alla jerkin' and just all of 'em alla jumpin' and sorta rockin and rollin' outta my own control, sorta.

Excerpt from Woody's play "My Forsaken Bibel." September 1956.

I played my "Songs to Grow On for Mother and Child" here for about 100 good patients and about 2 dozen good nurses and they all had so much fun they all want me to play my album again for them tomorrow morning. Amen. Amen.

–Woody's letter to his daughter "Puffy" (Nora Lee), October 15, 1956,

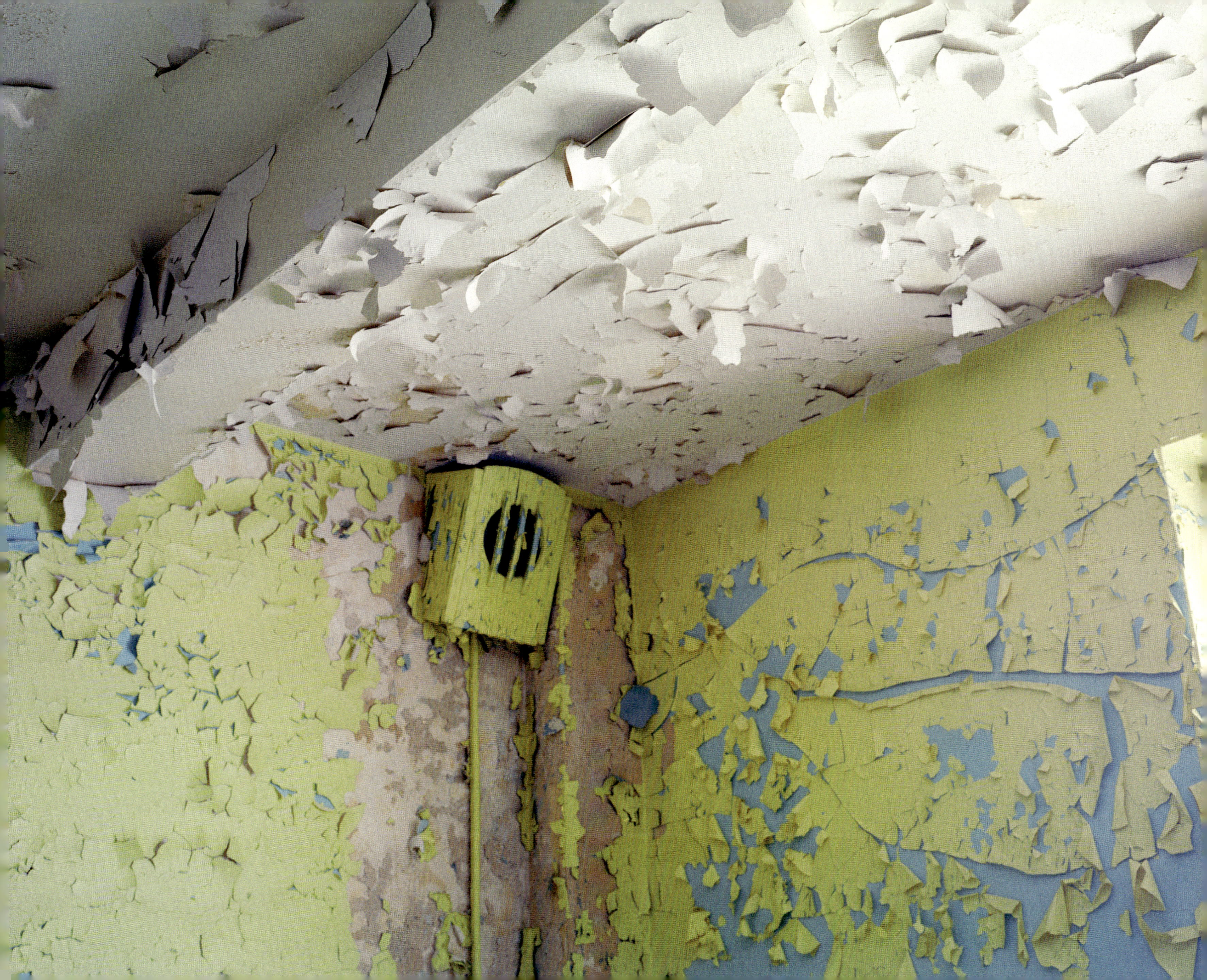

One time I brought out sheet music with his name on it, records, books, to show the head doctor. He said, "Well, Woody said he was a writer," and I would show him his book, and he didn't even look at it. "He said he wrote songs," and then I showed him the songs on the record and he ignored it all. Because, in the end, he's crazy. And Woody's remark to that was, "It's hard to tell who's the patient here." I did give some gratuities to the people that helped–the nurses, the personnel–and I told them more about his background.–*Harold Leventhal*

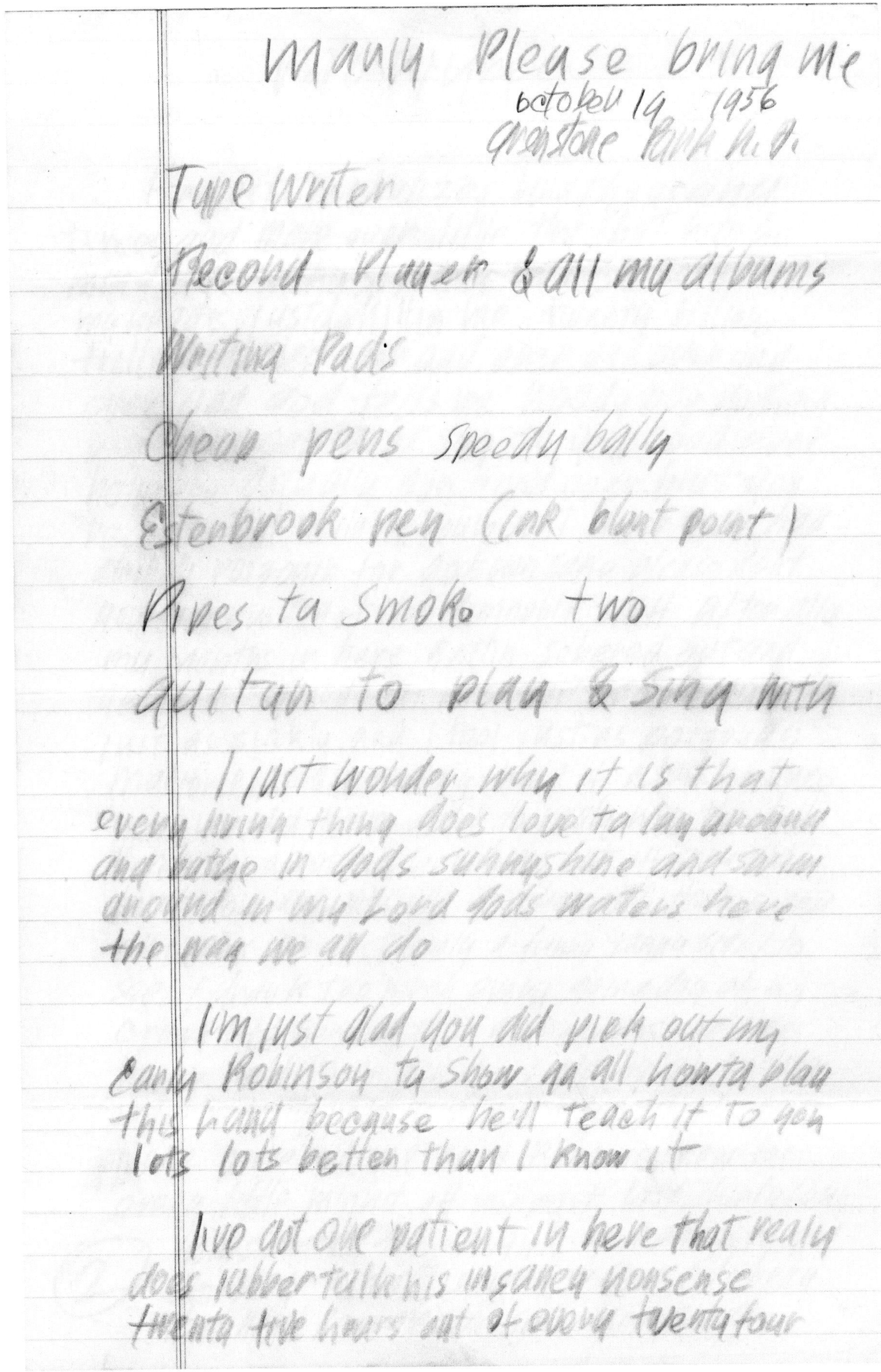
Marjy Please bring me
October 19 1956
Greystone Park N.J.

Type writer

Record Player & all my albums

Writing Pads

Cheap pens speedy ball

Esterbrook pen (ink blunt point)

Pipes ta smoke two

Guitar to play & sing with

I just wonder why it is that every living thing does love ta lay around and bathe in Gods sunnyshine and swim around in my Lord Gods waters here the way we all do

I'm just glad you did pick out my Early Robinson ta show ya all howta play this hand because he'll teach it to you lots lots better than I know it

I've got one patient in here that really does jabber talk his insaney nonsense twenty five hours out of every twenty four

Woody's letter to his wife, Marjorie. October 19, 1956.

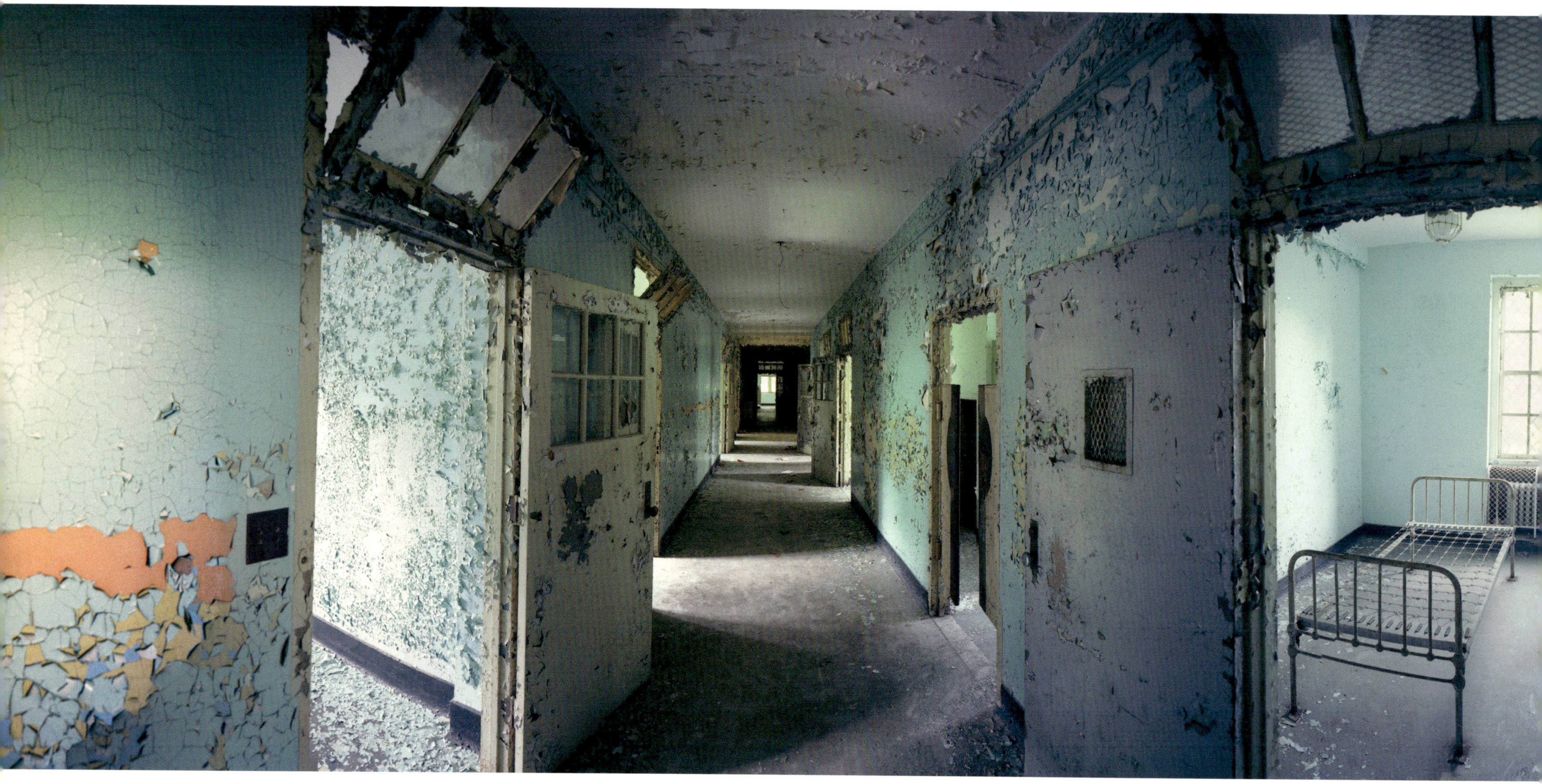

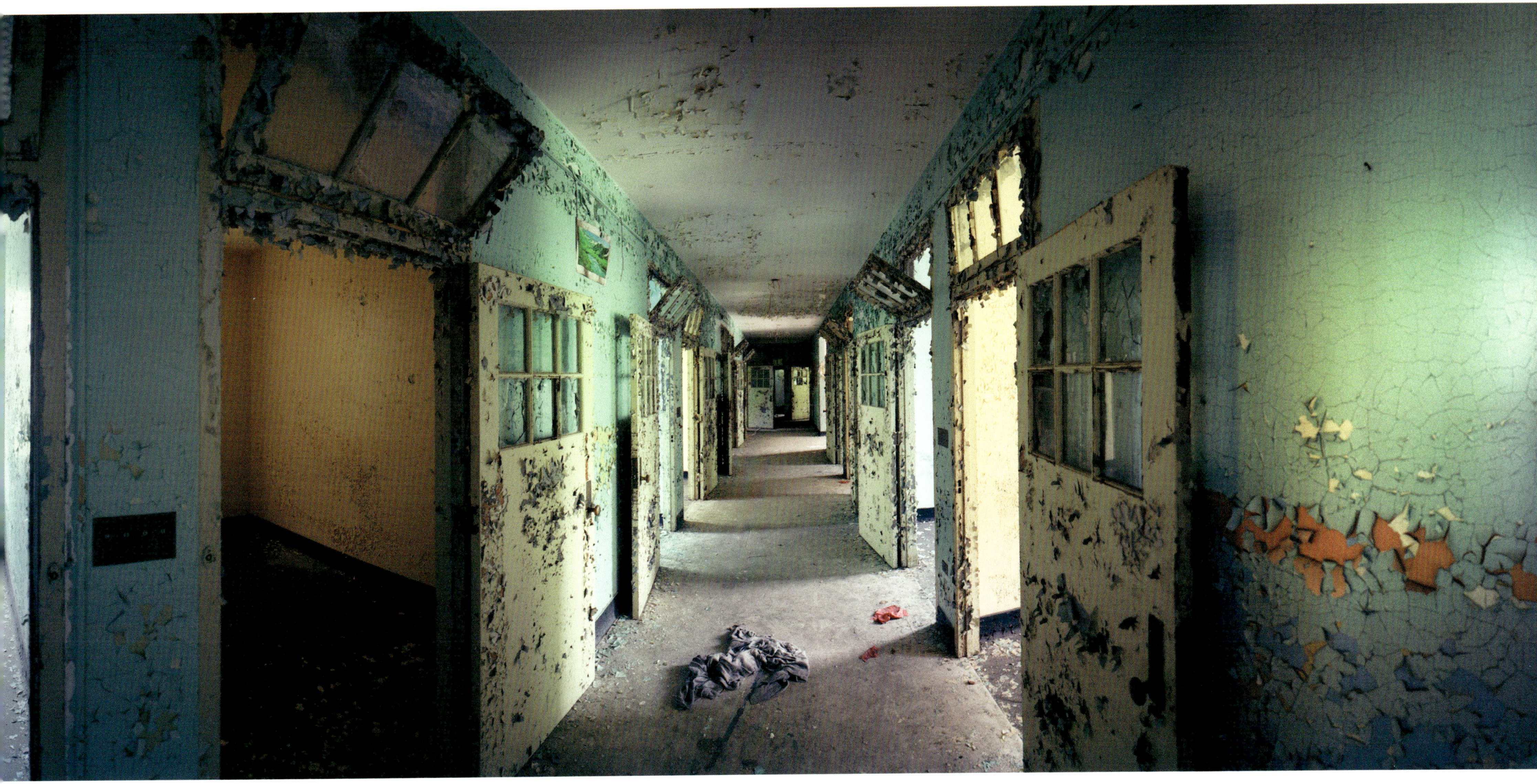

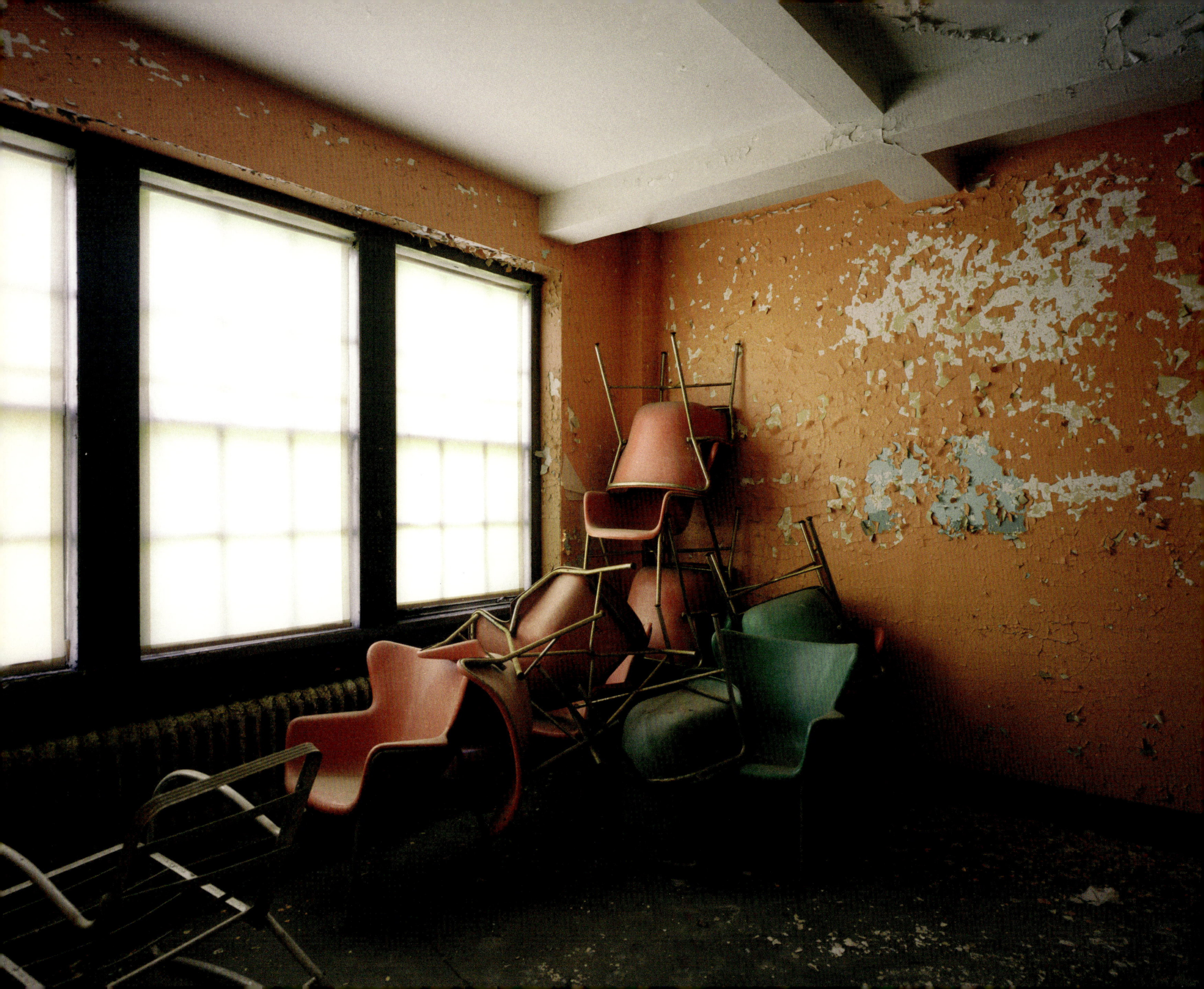

Dear Tinkin Jo

at 530am I wake up and slide my 30 chairs
back out of Pete's way so he cood sweep
and back again so he cood mop
I have to serve my 30 breakfasts at 7or715
and I help ta medicate alla them at 830
an read to my 30 my bible outloud from830 to 900
I make up ally our beds with Pete helpin me from 930 to 10
I help ta feed em all dinneroncemoreat 11or12-1230
I help ta medicate em all again from 3-30 pm
I serve em all their suppers after I unmake their beds

your blood brother

Woody

Woody's letter to his sister, Mary Jo. 1956

Joadeybunny

God is just giving me here
my real perfect kind of a chance
to just see and to just feel
exactly how my own Mother
saw and felt

amen agin

Woody

Woody's letter to his son, Joady. 1956.

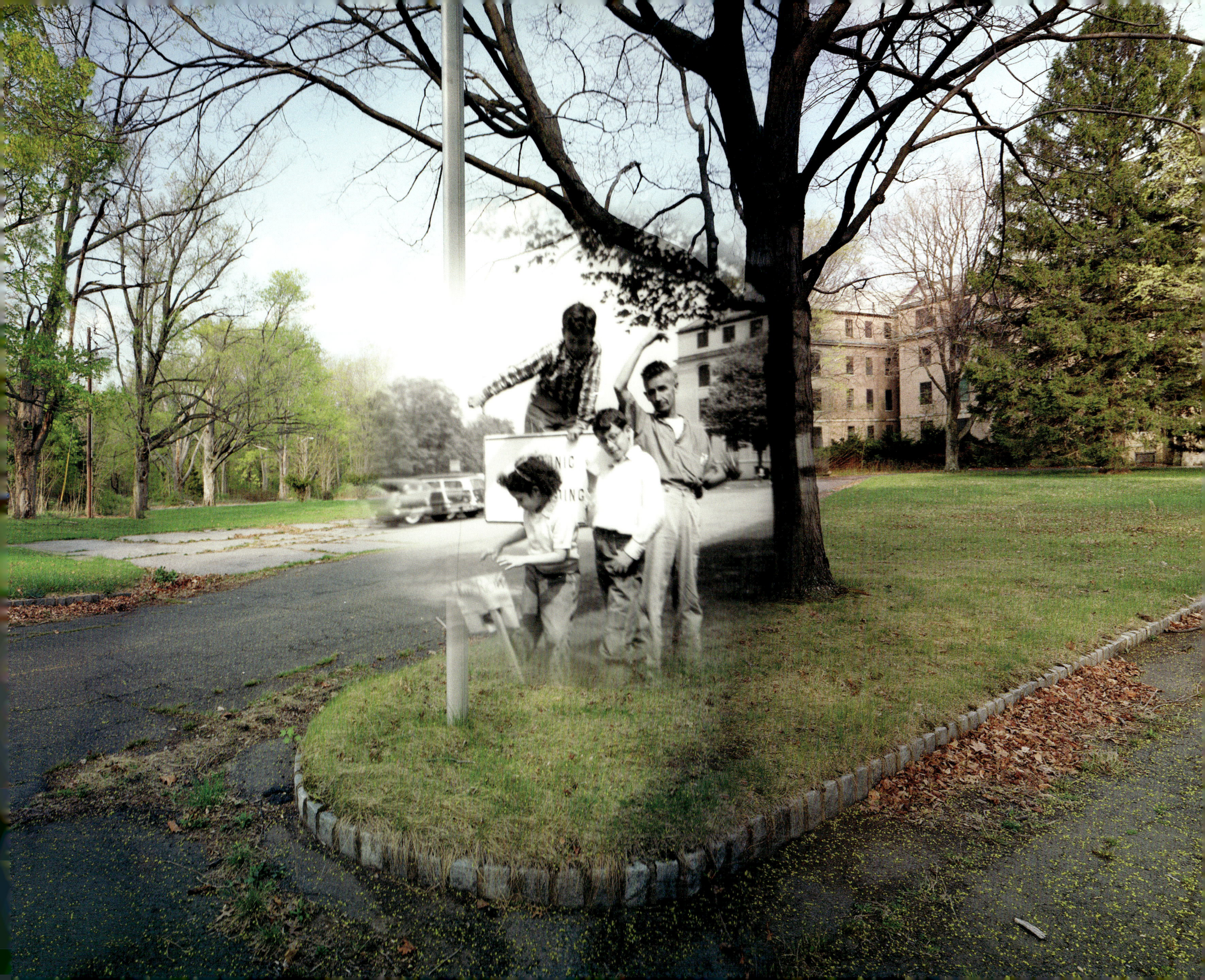

Sure, it was terrible. I tell you truly, my children only had Woody for a very short number of years when they were little. You know how kids scribble scrabble on paper? Woody would say, "Tell me what it's about," And then he would write under the scribble scrabble, "the moon is coming down, the rain is going up" or whatever the child said. There was a great respect for the child. When he first went into the hospital the children were 2, 3 and 4 and that short bit, whatever it was, was so great that it broke my heart that they couldn't have more because he was a wonderful father.

I'm sure that the children suffered in ways that I cannot describe because I couldn't speak for them. But we tried to maintain as much as we could of that joyousness that Woody had with kids. I remember a tree in front of one of the hospitals that we called the "Magiky Tree". . .

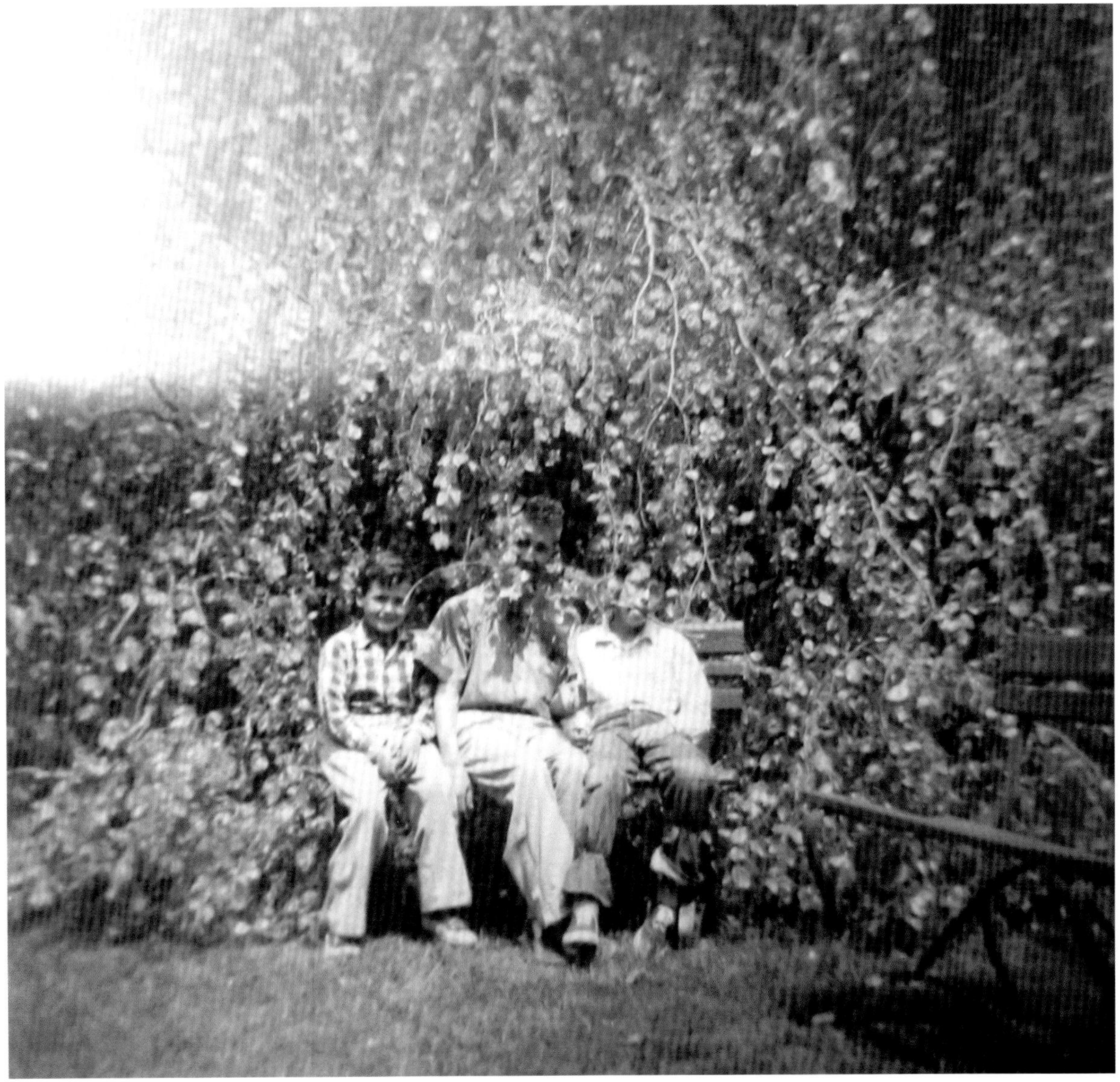

Joady, Woody, and Arlo under the "Magiky Tree." 1959.

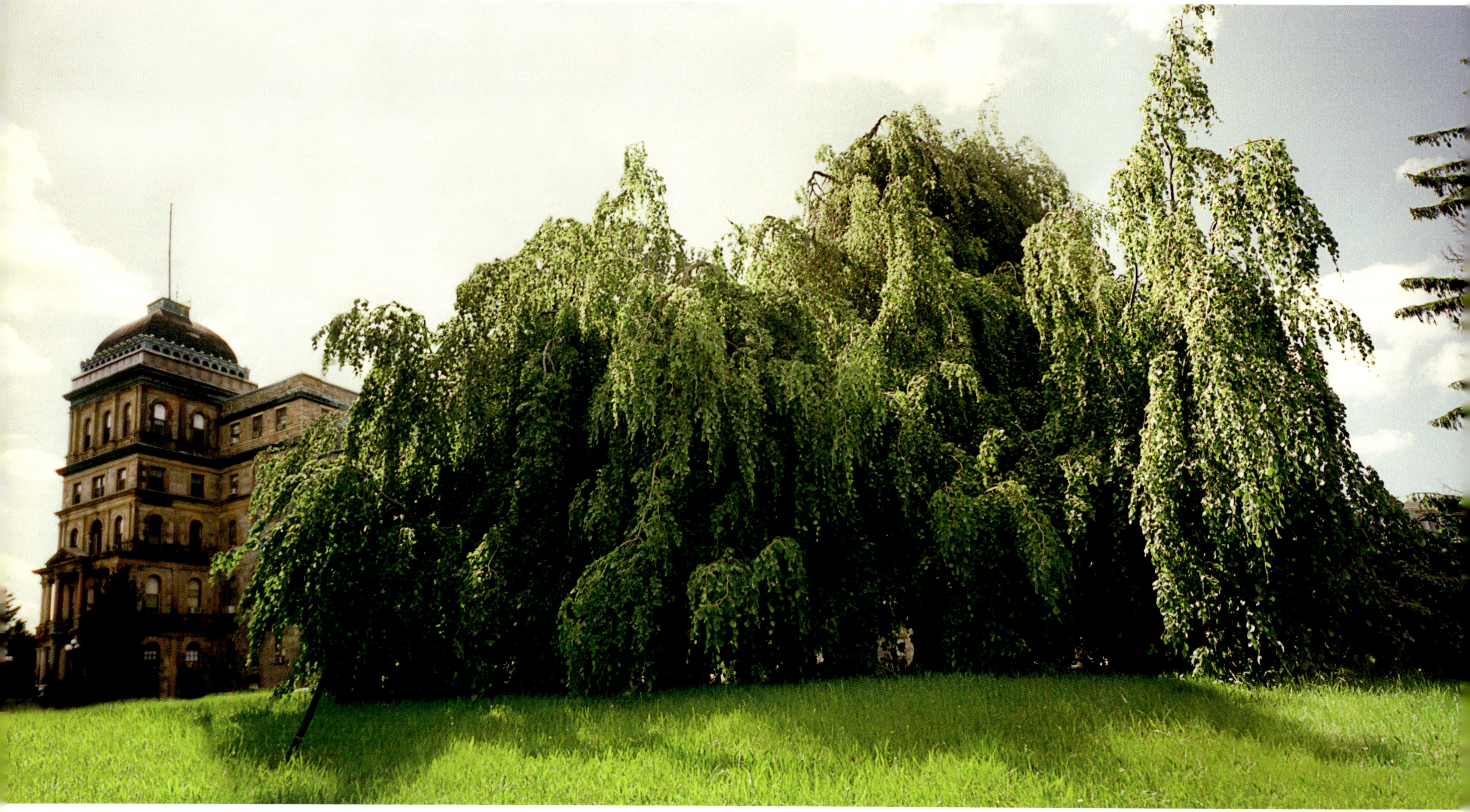

the branches go way out and touch the ground so it sort of creates a tent. So I would have the children wait under the "Magiky Tree" while I'd go to get Woody and bring him down and then we'd make a picnic out of it. So I tried to make the visits in the hospital like a fun day.

When we would go to a restaurant and Woody would drop and slip and slurp all the things because of the involuntary movement, people would stare at us, and I would say, out loud, so there's no question about it, "Oh, Woody's sick today. He sure is." And we'd just make a joke about it. And just laugh, and he would laugh, you know, "Yep."–*Marjorie Guthrie*

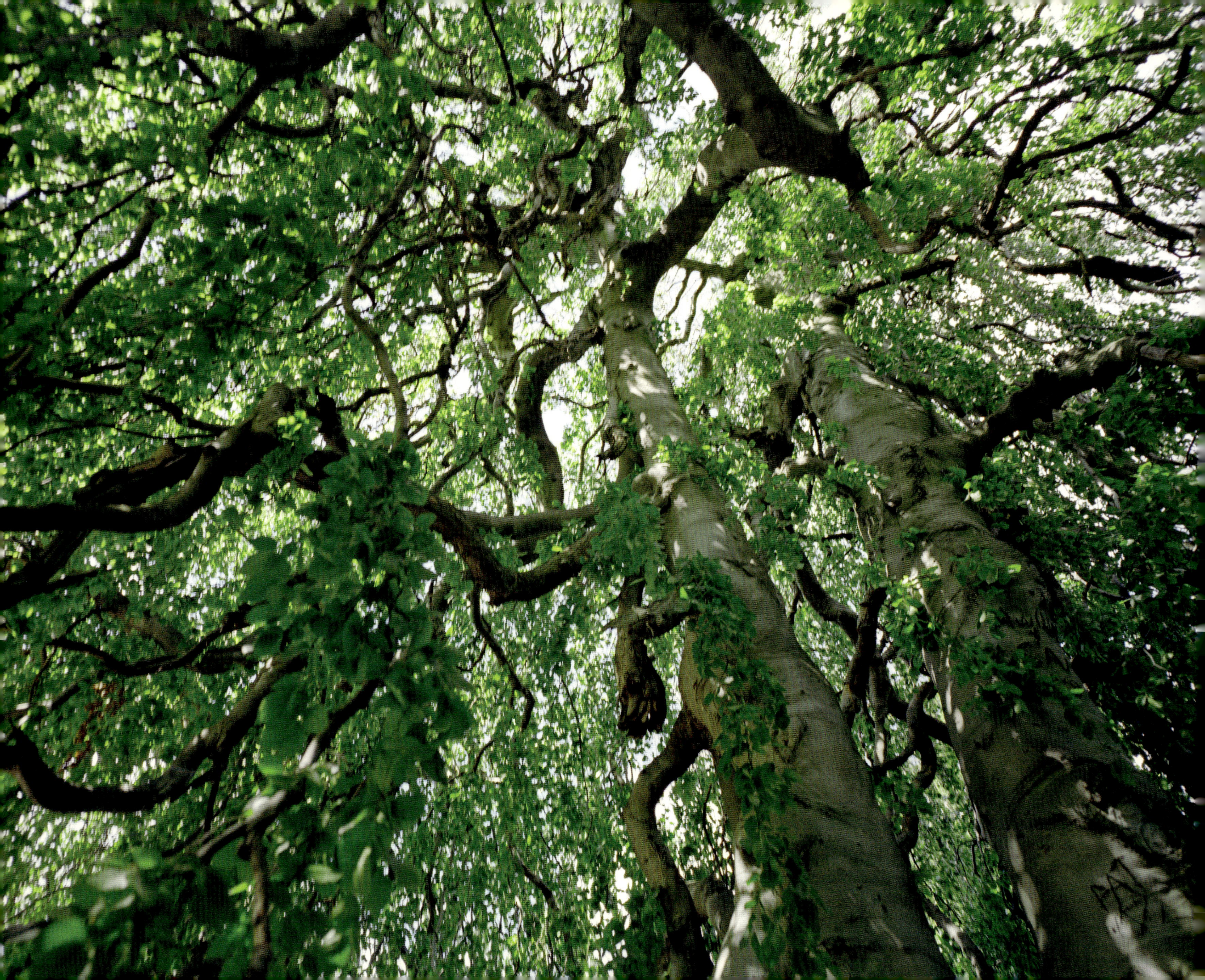

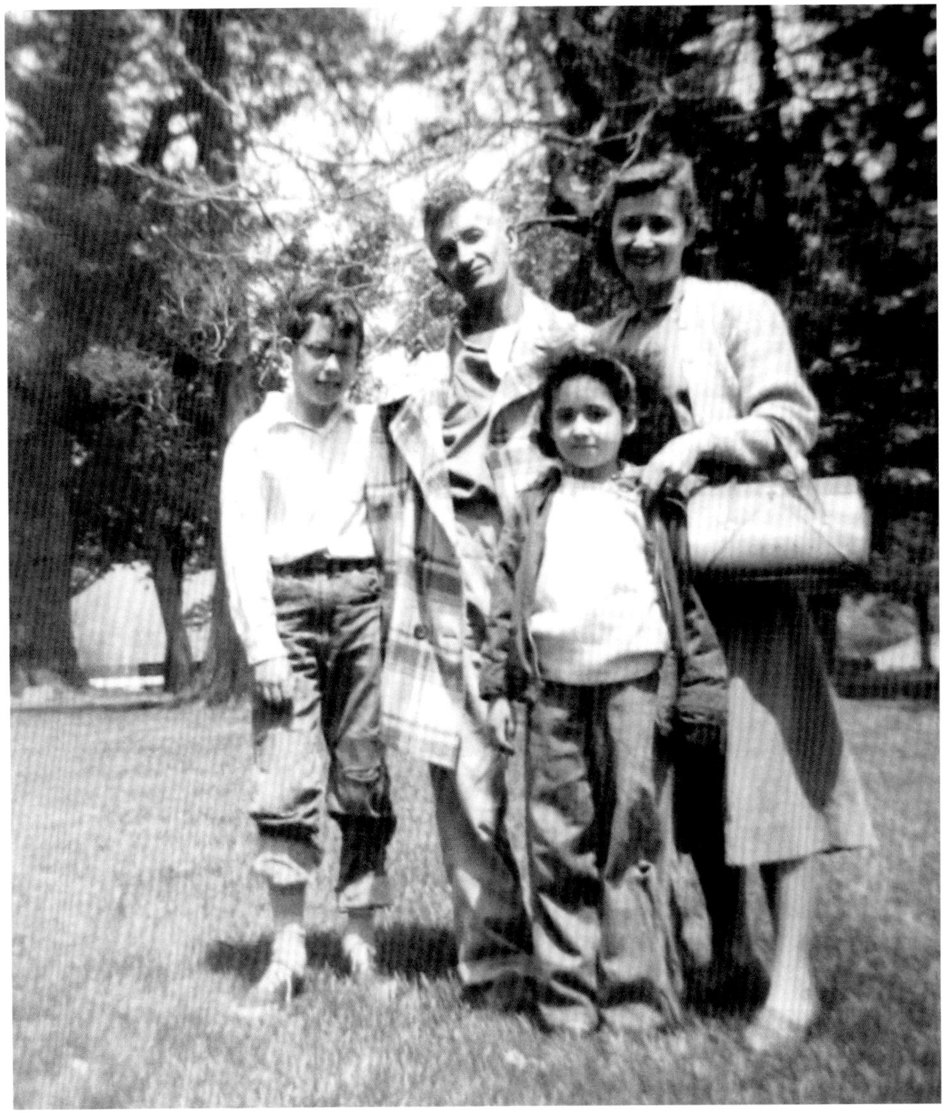

Arlo, Woody, Nora Lee, and Marjorie. 1959.

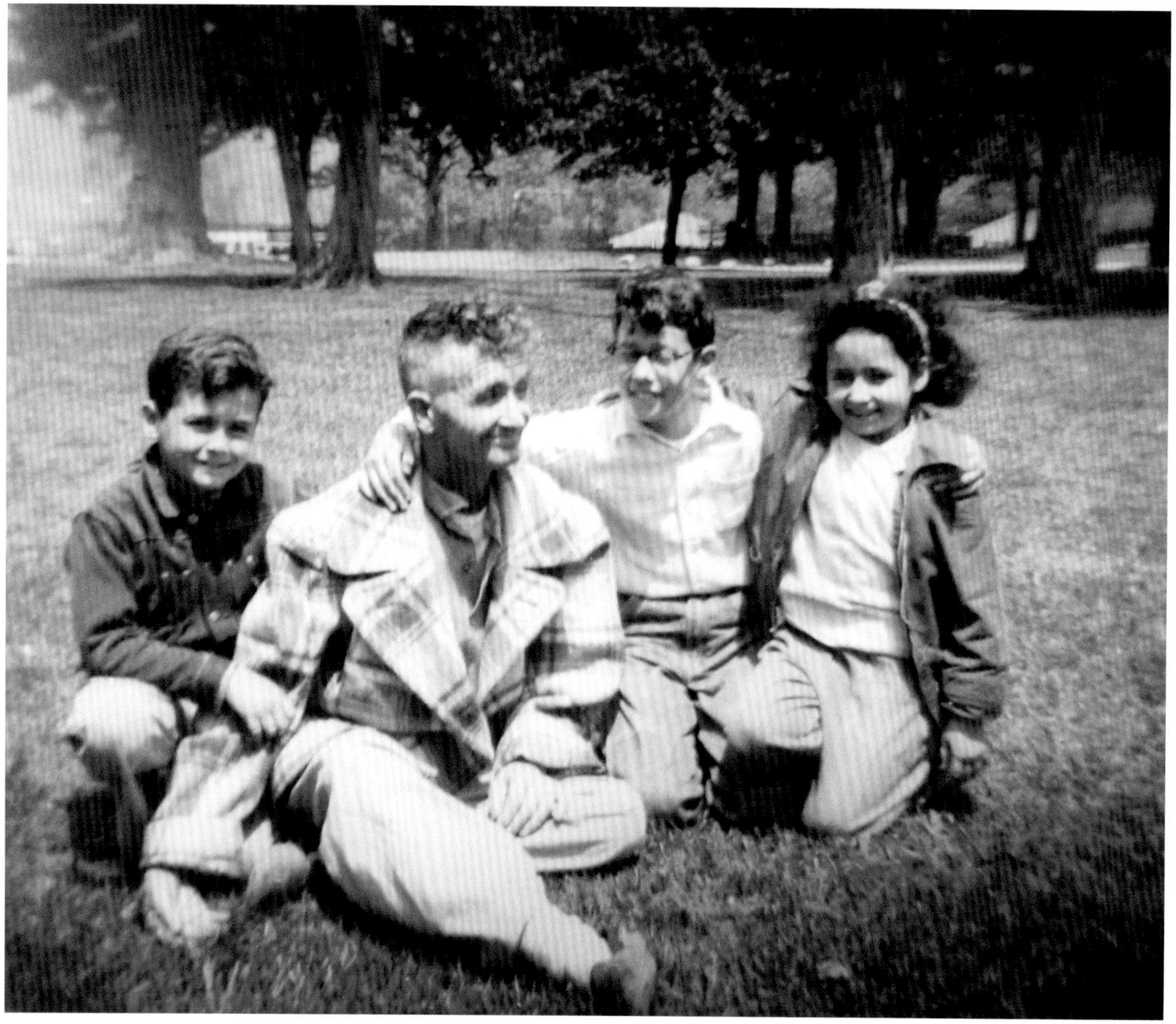

Joady, Woody, Arlo, and Nora Lee. 1959.

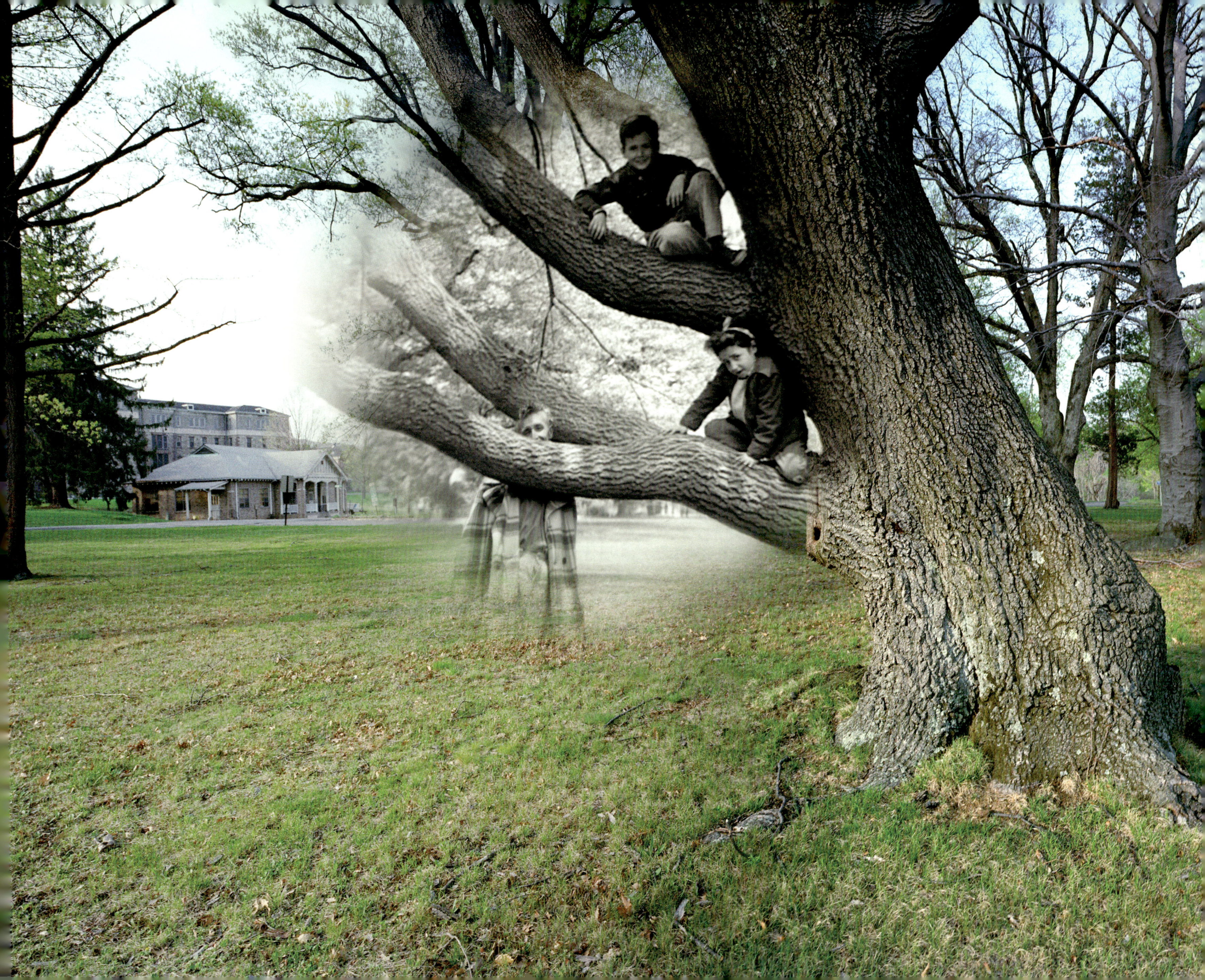

Most Sundays we would drive out to Greystone Hospital to visit my father. It was a long drive from Howard Beach, Queens to Morris Plains, New Jersey. When all the other kids were off from school, we would pile into the car for this emotionally and physically draining journey. We drove along the Belt Parkway into Manhattan, through the Holland or the Lincoln Tunnel, and onto the New Jersey highways. This took us to the long, dramatic driveway entering the hospital grounds. That's when I felt the fear coming. The grounds were enormous. We were entering a city filled with patients and their families, nurses and doctors.–*Nora Guthrie*

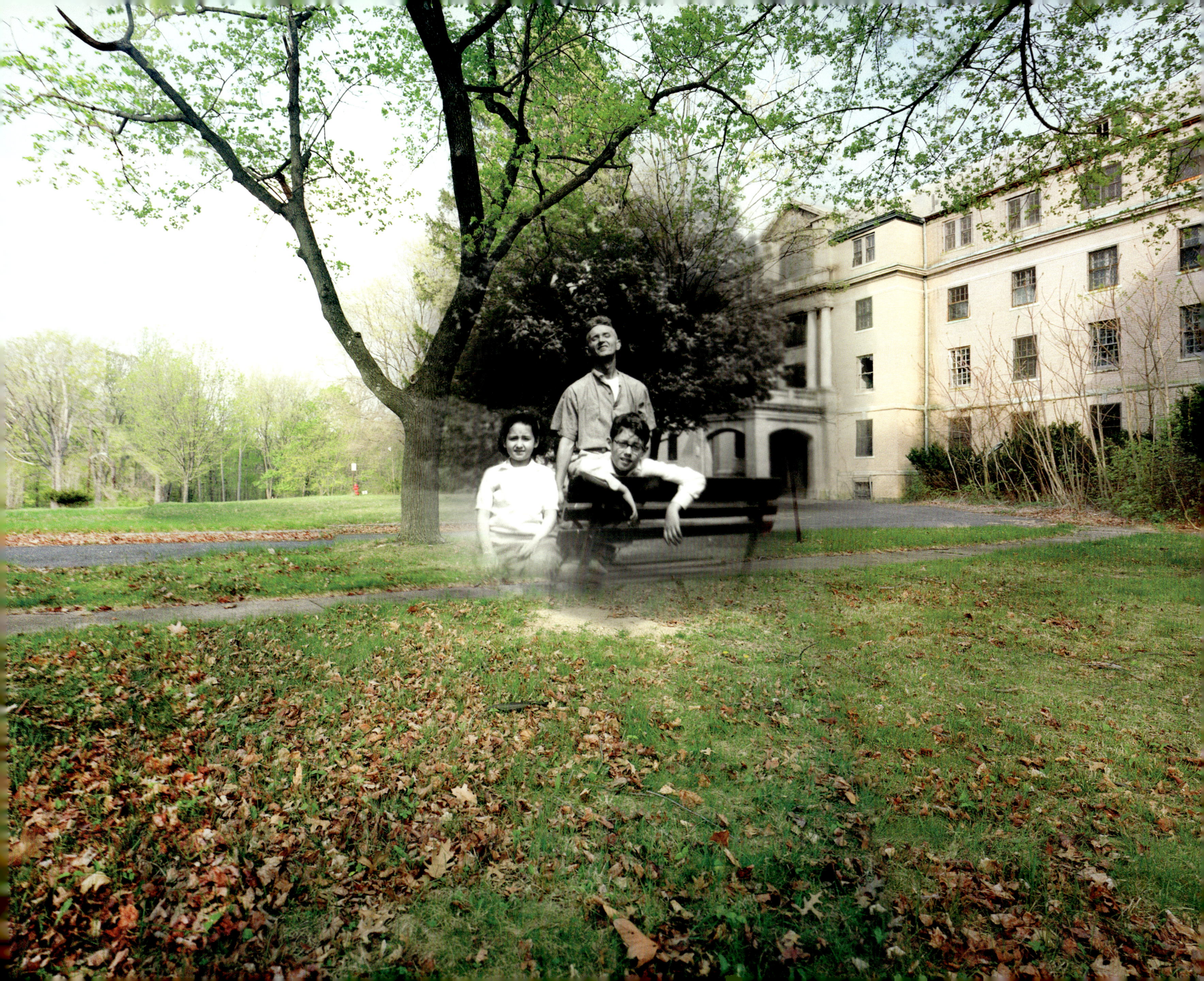

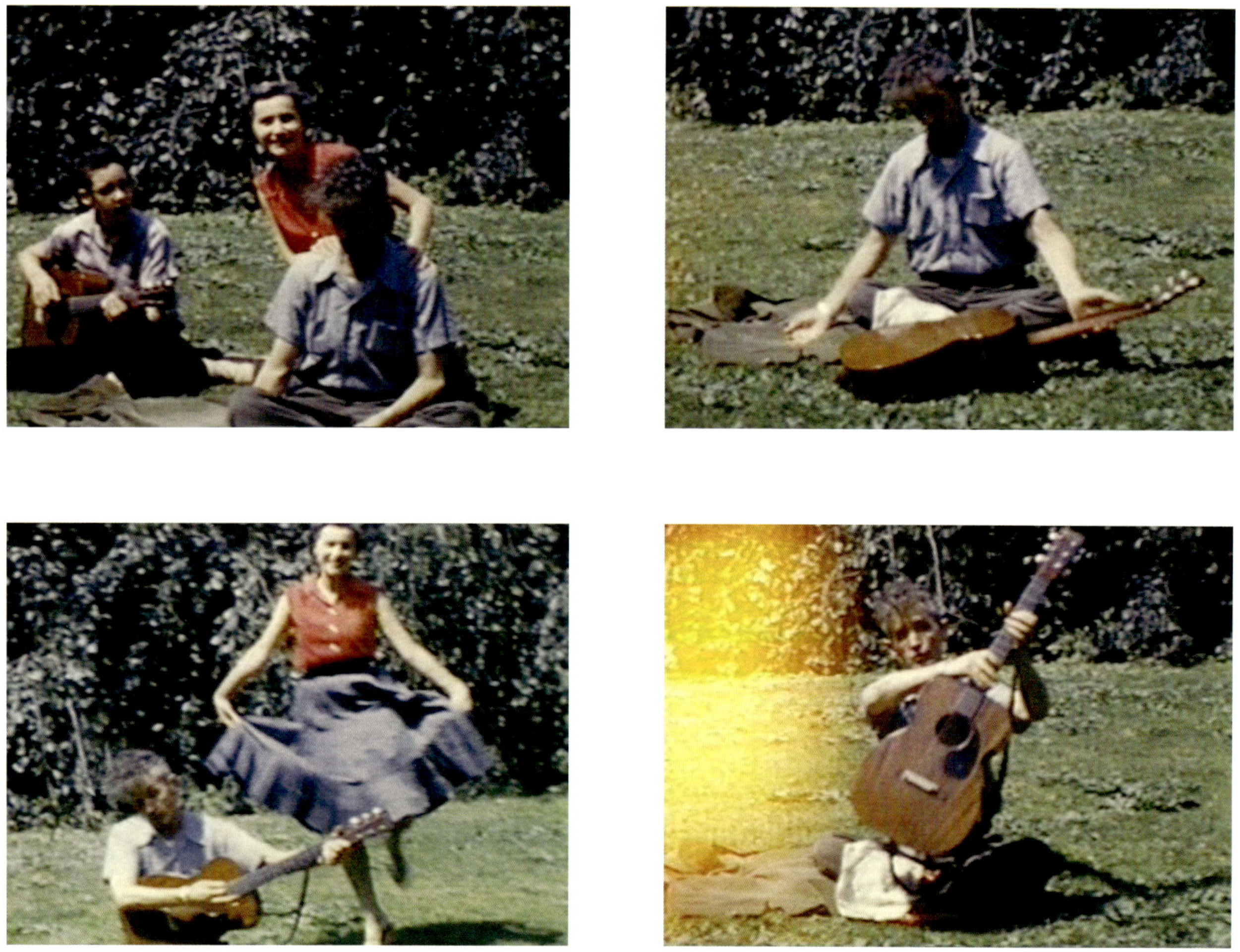

Arlo, Marjorie, and Woody. 1960.

Deary Arlo Davy

I wanta goatt here and climb up my
magiky tree with you all
the very next old time you all
come here to visit me

Gotta sleep
daddy me

Woody Guthrie

Decembre once more
1956

Woody's letter to his son, Arlo. 1956.

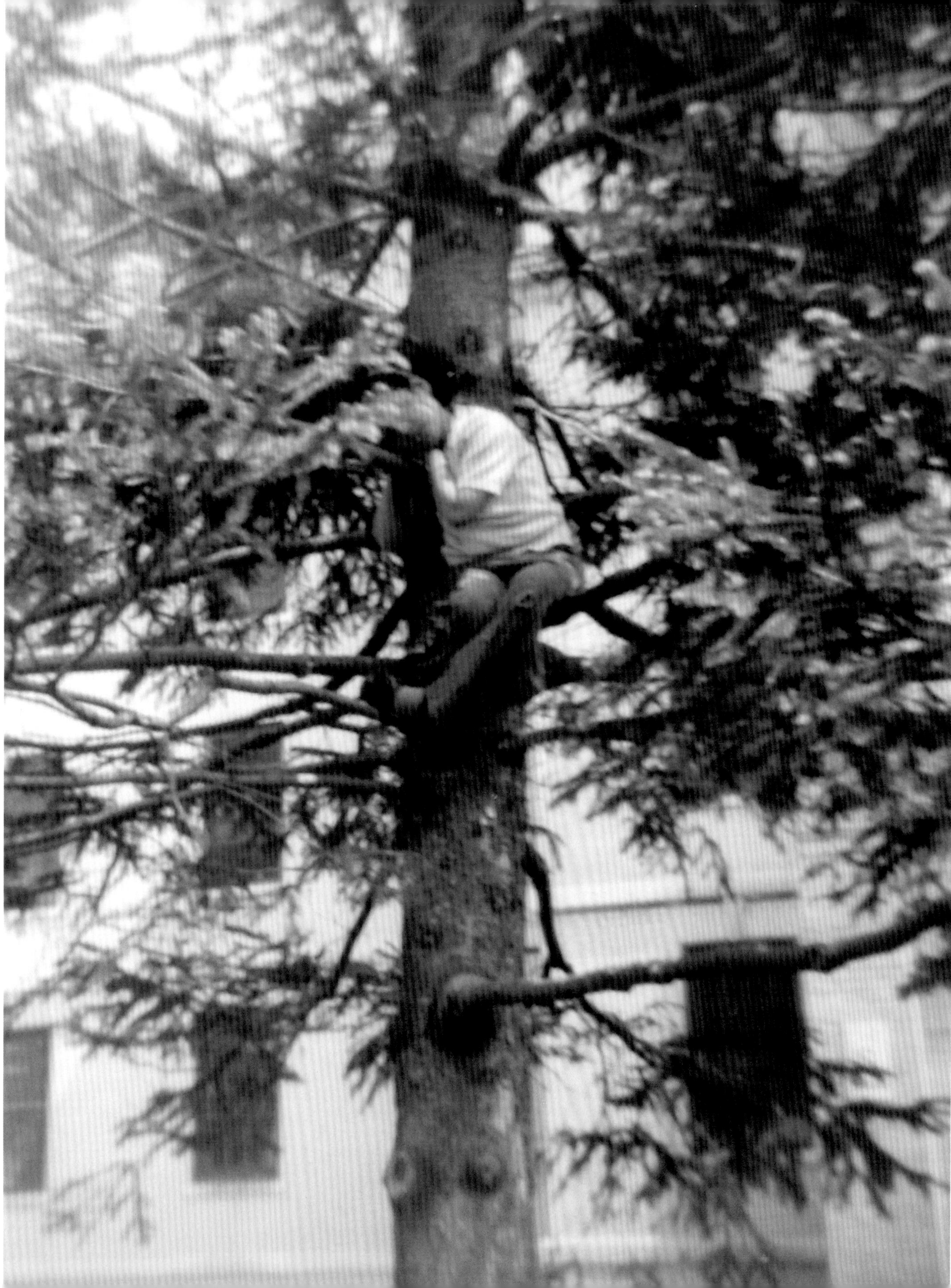

Nora Lee. 1959.

At some point or other, we'd take my dad out of there. We took him from Greystone over to people's homes in the area. And we would play music and we would goof off and we would try to integrate him in the world that was celebrating the very things that he thought was important. I mean, his work was booming as he entered Greystone. And I think my mom really wanted him to understand and participate in it to some extent, as much as he could. And that's what we did. That was our life.*–Arlo Guthrie*

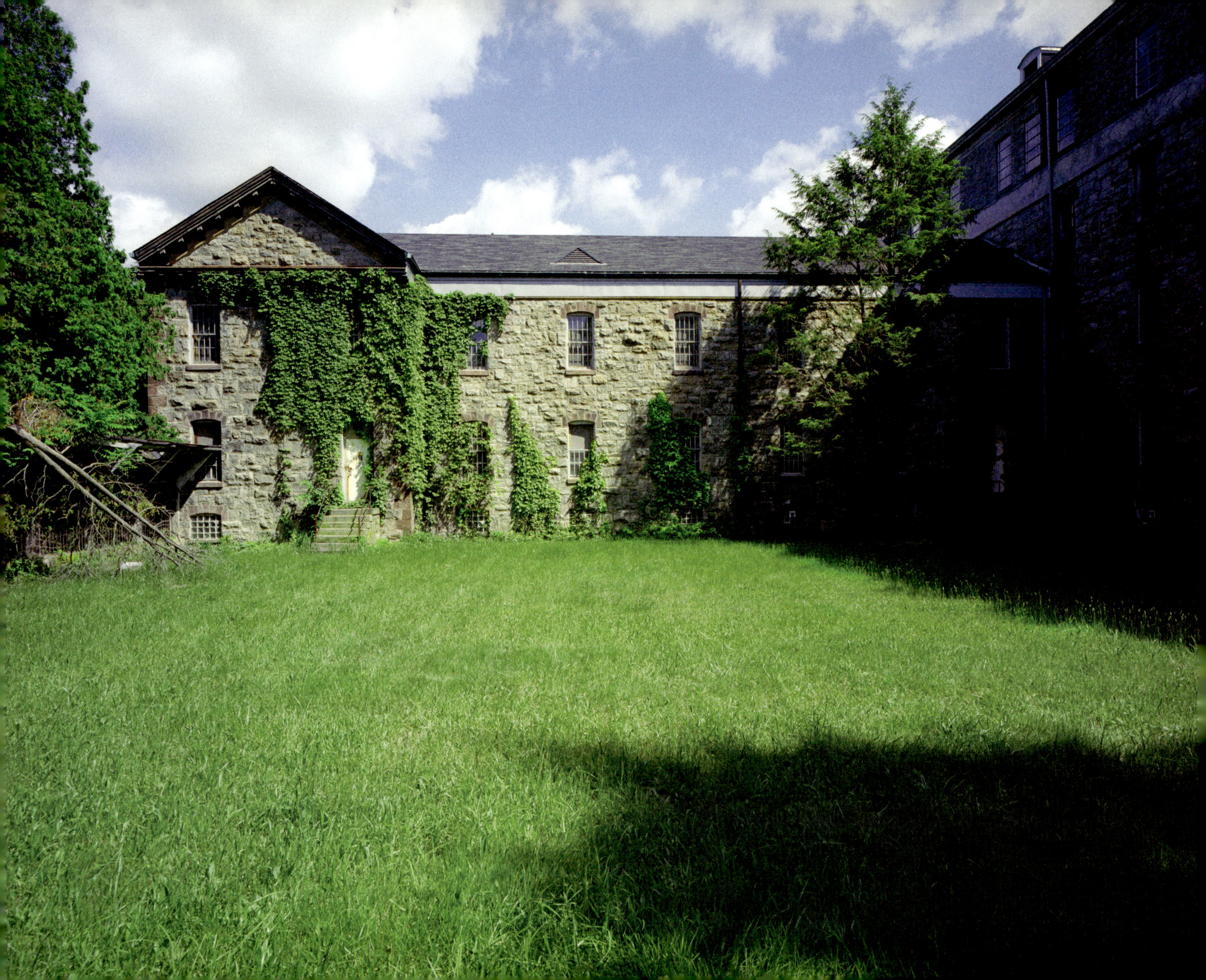

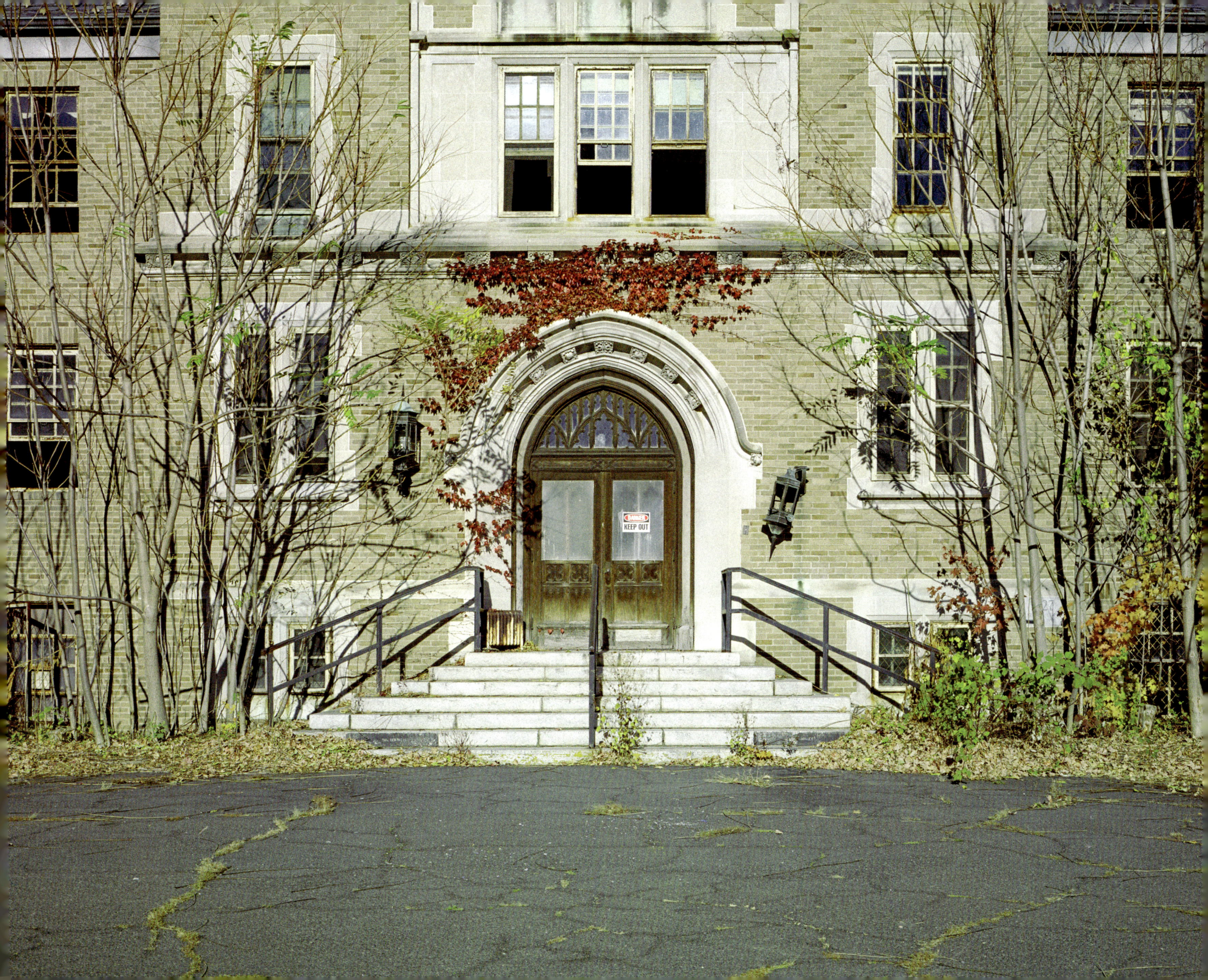
KEEP OUT

e Youre doin to

realy goody Artisty Painter

I See lotsa good

good pitcures handpainted

hungup here along alla my

Greystoney Hospital walls

Love Me

daddy Weeds

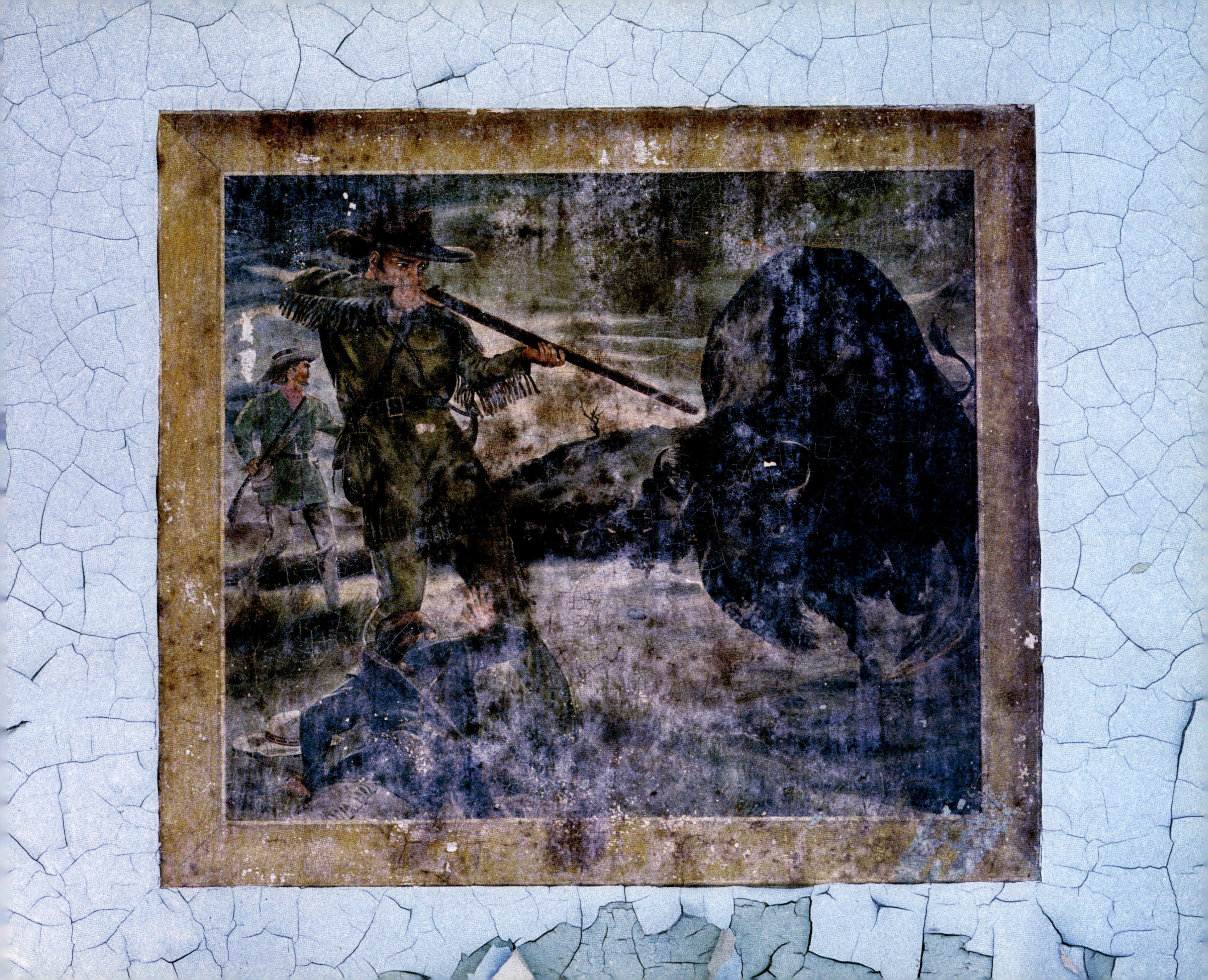

He bought Arlo his first guitar on his sixth birthday. Woody had been in and out of the hospital already. Arlo had always made believe he was playing guitar, you know how kids do when you'd see your father do something. When Woody became ill I wanted the kids to play. I didn't know how to play, I always played the piano, so I went and got a little book—I was determined I was going to take Woody's place after all the music was gone. I taught Arlo a C chord and a G chord and with a few little things like that he got started. And of course, later Arlo always played for Woody at the hospital.

"Alice's Restaurant" came out the very year that Woody died. Right before he died I went to the hospital with the brochure announcing Arlo singing at Carnegie Hall and I just said, "Well look at this, look who's singing in Carnegie Hall, not Woody Guthrie, Arlo Guthrie." The two of us got such a kick out it. Woody never sang in Carnegie Hall. He sang in a union hall where everybody was blowing their noses and talking while he was singing.

—Marjorie Guthrie

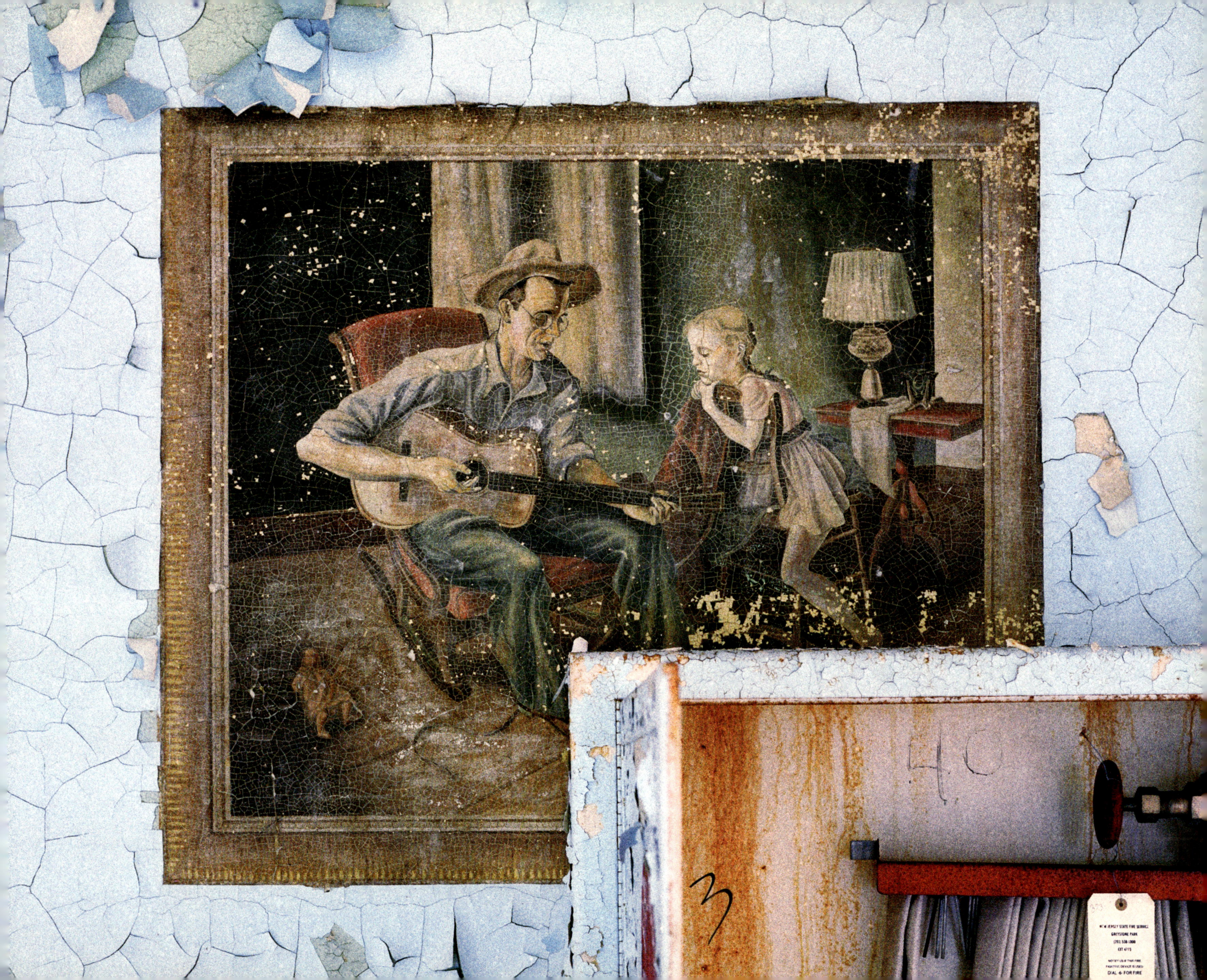
NEW JERSEY STATE FIRE SERVICE
GREYSTONE PARK
DIAL 6 FOR FIRE

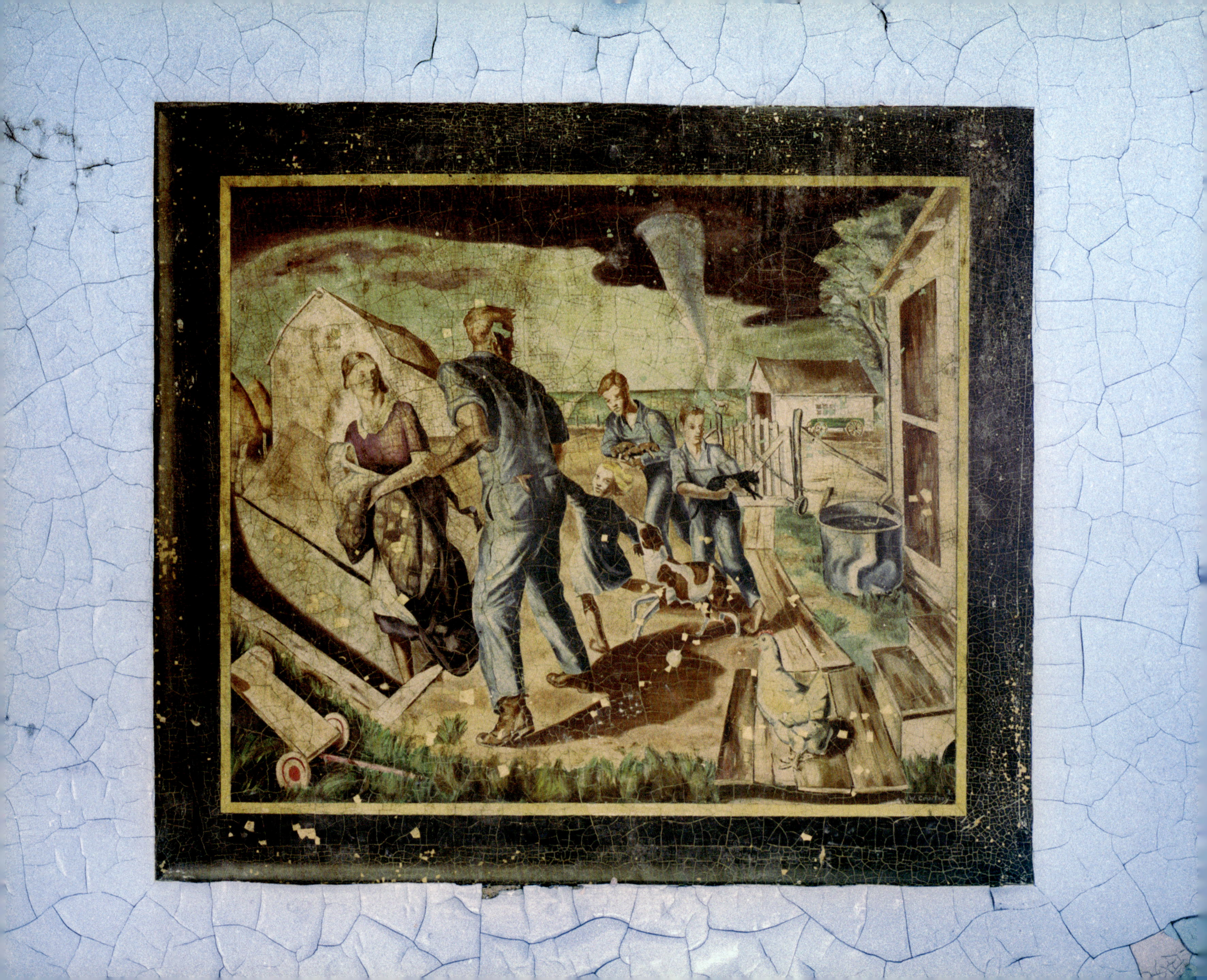

Deary Marjyree

Ya can go tell mister Eisendyhower
that he cant be my big chiefy bossy man
till he makes alla my untied states
allamy races all equal

I'll save my vote here
for my communist candidates anyhow
that'll be my onlyest ones
ta ever even partlyways try ta give birth
ta my racey equality

lovey me write
daddy Woody

Woody's letter to his wife, Marjorie. 1956.

And the sad part, really, is that Woody spent all those years in a state hospital because it was presumed that he was going to be a vegetable at the end of his life. He never did become a vegetable. He looked like a vegetable—he couldn't walk, he couldn't talk, his involuntary movement was hard to control—but when I came to visit I could see by the laughter or the look on his face that he enjoyed what I was saying or doing.

Finally, right near the end in 1967, those last couple of months, I began to call Dr. Wittier over to the bedside and I would say, "Dr. Wittier, Woody is not a vegetable, he knows everything I'm saying." I made three cards, a "yes," a "no," and a "question mark" and I spread them out on the bed and I said, "Woody, let's show Dr. Wittier that you know everything I'm talking about." And I asked him questions to which I knew the answer. And he would make a face at me as if to say, "You know I was born in Okemah," and I said, "Yes, I know I know, but I want Dr. Wittier to see that you know and that your memory is still functioning." And Woody kept showing me that although his memory wasn't perfect, he was still a whole person. But he looked awful. And imagine what it was like, having a functioning brain and living with 44 men who were mentally incompetent.—*Marjorie Guthrie*

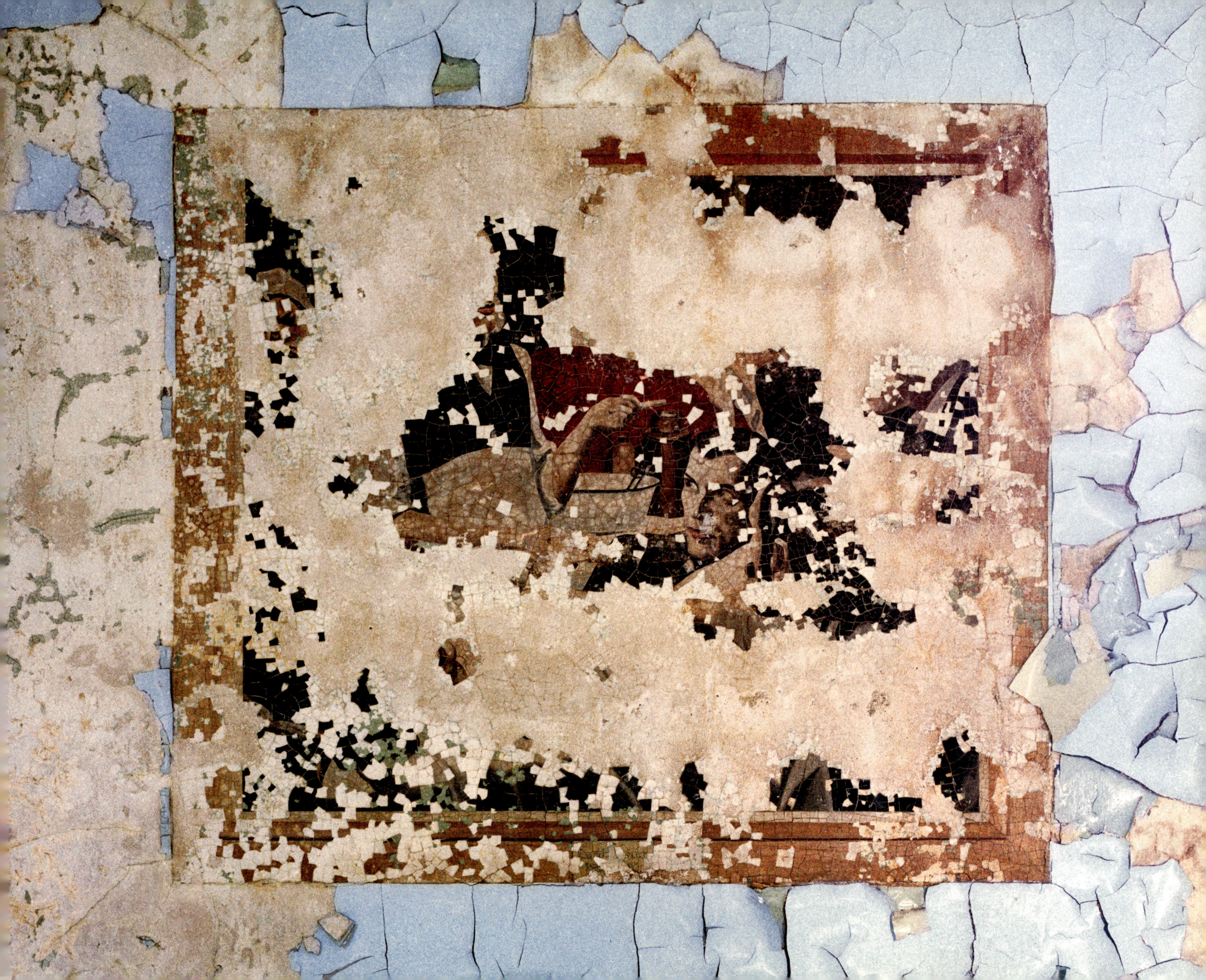

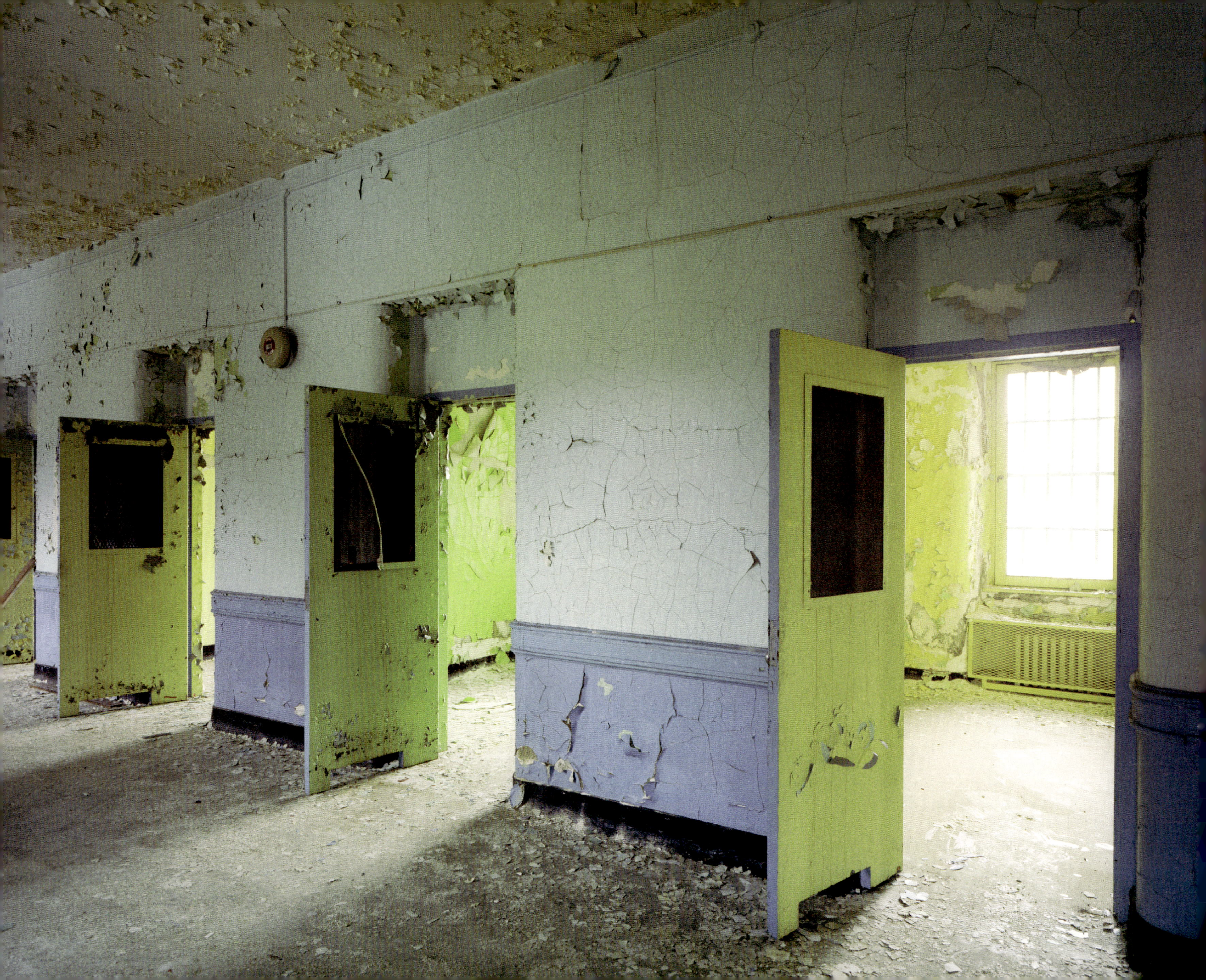

To us, it was just a normal thing. My dad was in the hospital, and we would go see him. I understood that he was sick, and it was clearly visible. Over the years, of course, as I got older, I knew more and more about it, and was actually responsible for him to some extent. As I said, when I went back recently, it wasn't any different. You know how sometimes you go back to a place and it seems smaller? Greystone didn't seem any smaller. It seemed exactly the same.–*Arlo Guthrie*

What's kind of nice is that I remember Bob Dylan and John Cohen. I can't quite remember all of them, but we used to meet in our very dear friends' home in New Jersey, the Gleasons, a lovely couple. And Woody would want to touch the guitar and play it and his hands were uncontrolled and he couldn't play it well from the Huntington's Chorea, so he would just sort of hold it lovingly and strum it very awkwardly, but the other kids would all play the music, so he felt like he was still part of it.–*Marjorie Guthrie*

I knew him (Woody) before I went back East [likely 1936]. We were out in Arizona and there's a big river along here, and we were building that [Hoover] dam. I was baking bread and biscuits. I heard this guitar playing and I walked to where the guitar was, and there was Woody. Woody traveled all over the country. He went here and he went there, and he went someplace else and he always took his guitar with him. I went over and started talking to him, and he said, "Well, right now I don't know which way I'm gonna go, but one of these days I'll probably end up at your front door"—and that is exactly what happened a number of years afterwards.—*Sidsel Gleason*

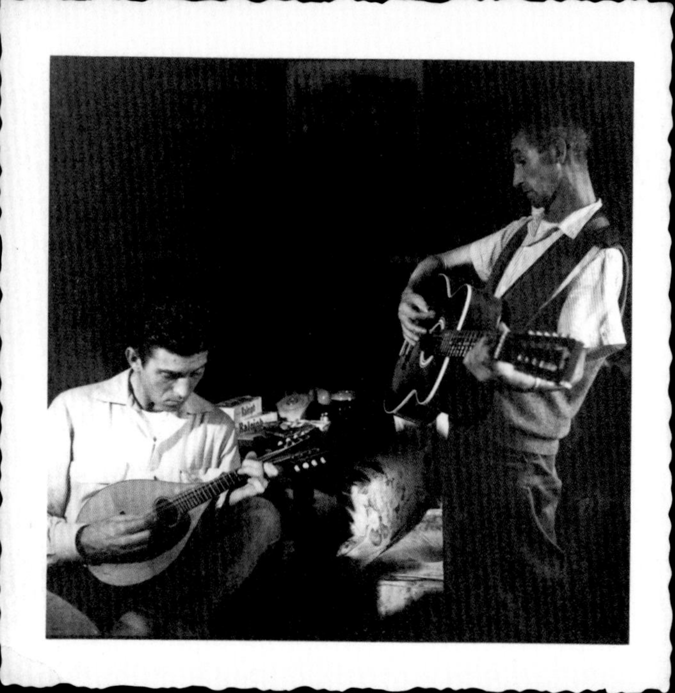

Ernie Marrs and Woody at Pete Seeger's home. 1961.

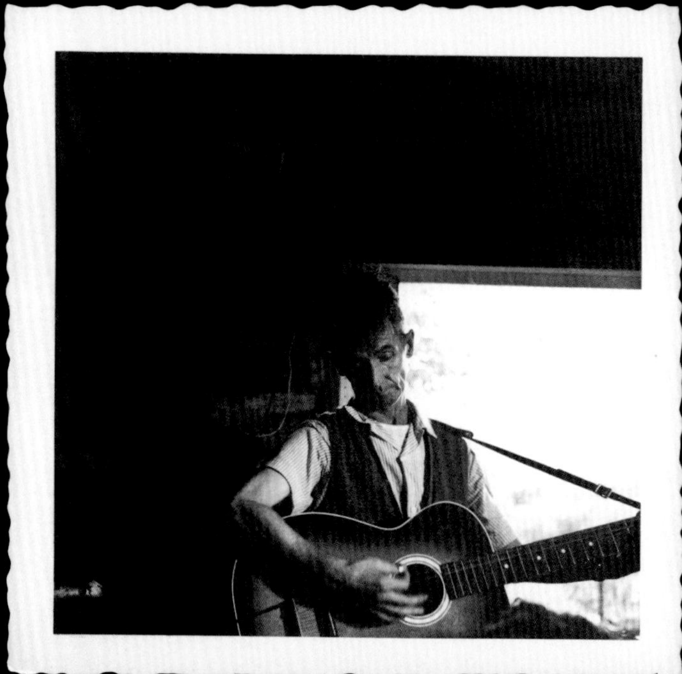

My husband got permission to take him off of the grounds, which was unbelievable that he got him off there. And we went up to get him every Sunday, just like clockwork. I had to make cowboy stew and biscuits for him. I had a great big cast iron kettle. And he said, "I would crawl clear out from there for your cowboy stew, I love it." And every week we'd go out and get him. He'd always say, "Biscuits this time?" "Yup." "Okay," he'd say. –*Sidsel Gleason*

I can't remember why I went there or what gave me the impetus to go get him. But I know that he needed to get out of there. I had that feeling. I remember the feeling of going to the back entrance, sort of a lobby there. I'd say, "I want to visit with Woody Guthrie." I'd stand there in the lobby and see all of these old men just kind of wandering aimlessly about, sitting here and there. I didn't know what he would look like at that time. And that he emerged from that place is very moving and challenging to me. I just felt that I wanted to bring some enjoyment into that life, and bring him to these concerts or bring him into Washington Square, to see what was happening. But I don't know what got me off my ass to make that bold move.*–John Cohen*

John Cohen, and Woody at the Gleason's home. 1960.

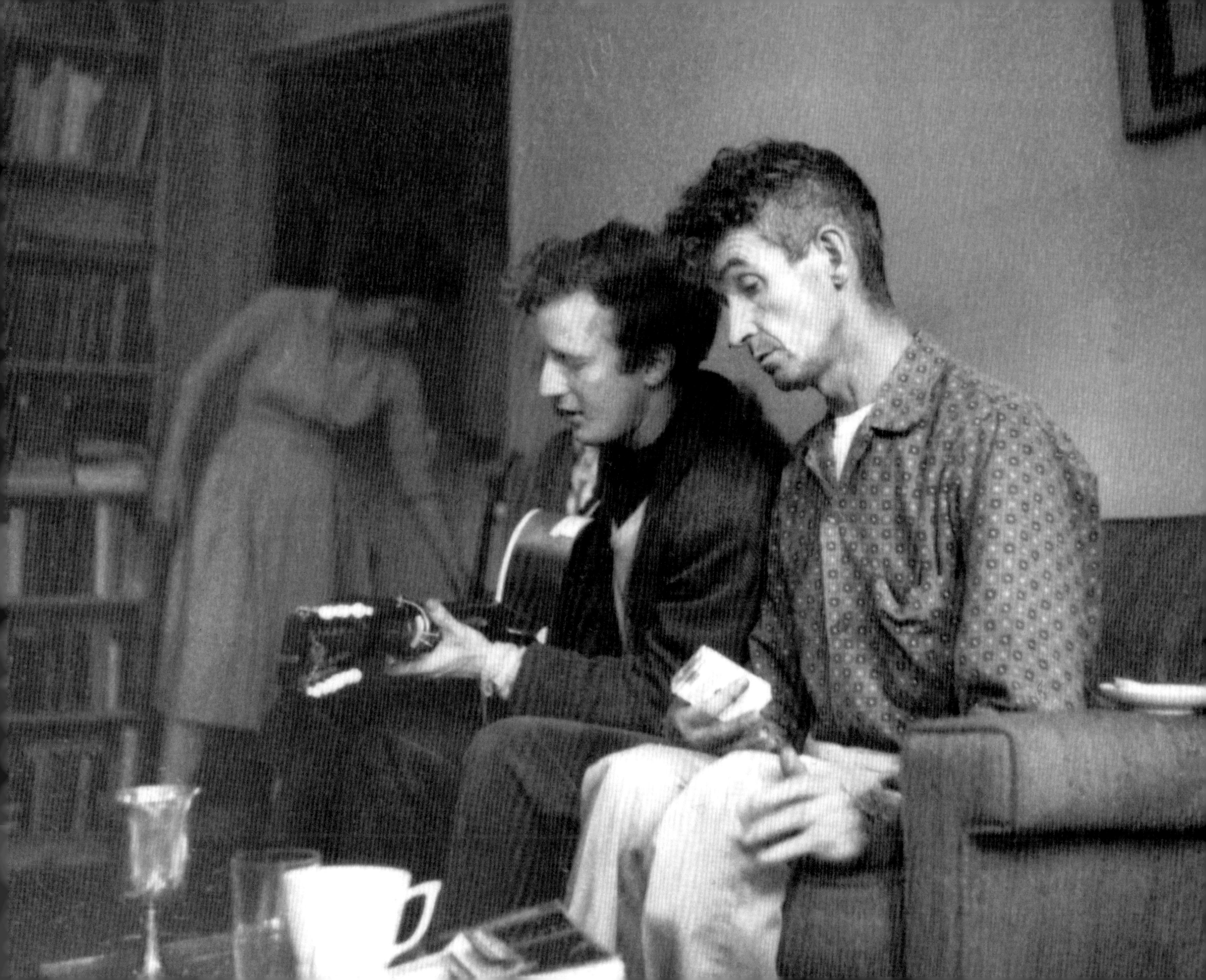

I think I must have gone to the Gleason's maybe a total of two or three times with him. And one of those times, I was out there at the same time Jack came back to the States, and he was seeing Woody after all his years in England. I thought there was something special about it. It was simply interesting to have this guy who was carrying on Woody's songs and Woody's character while Woody was sort of being shut down in Greystone.–*John Cohen*

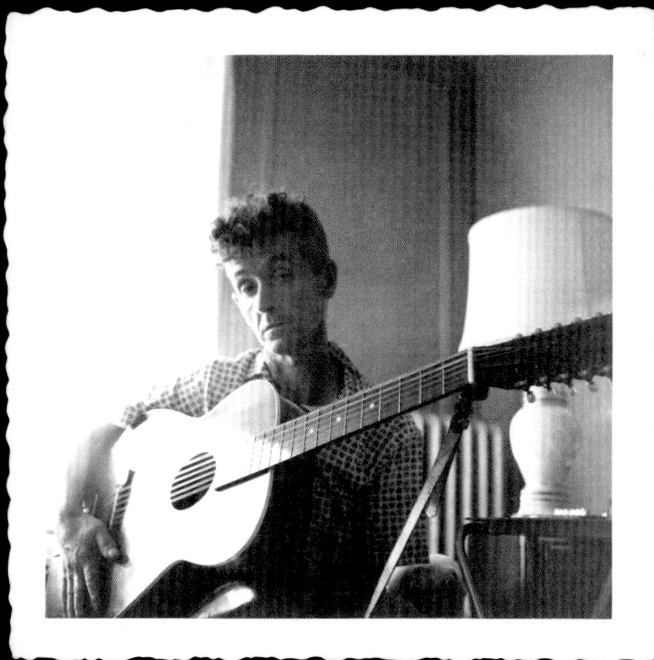

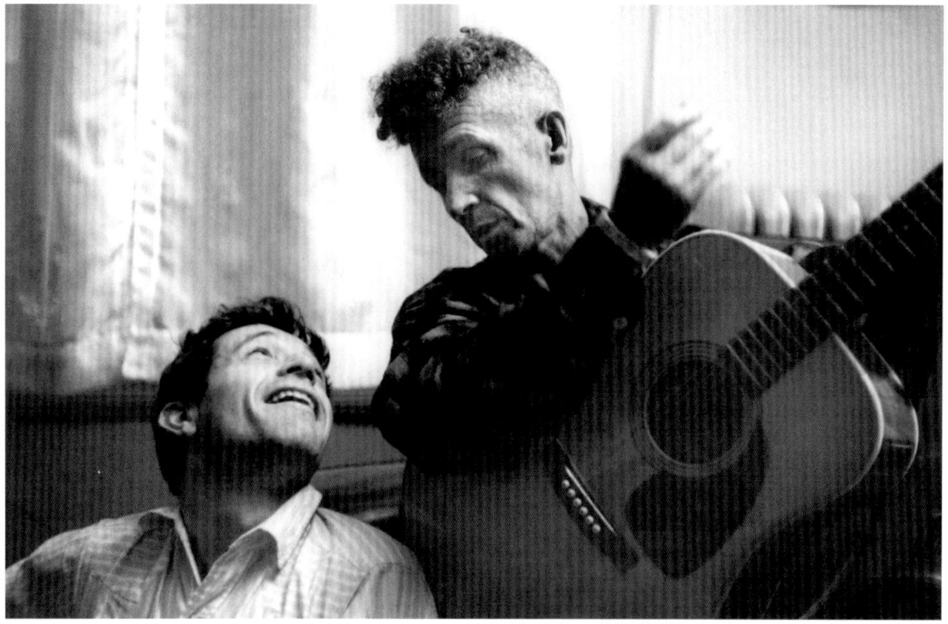 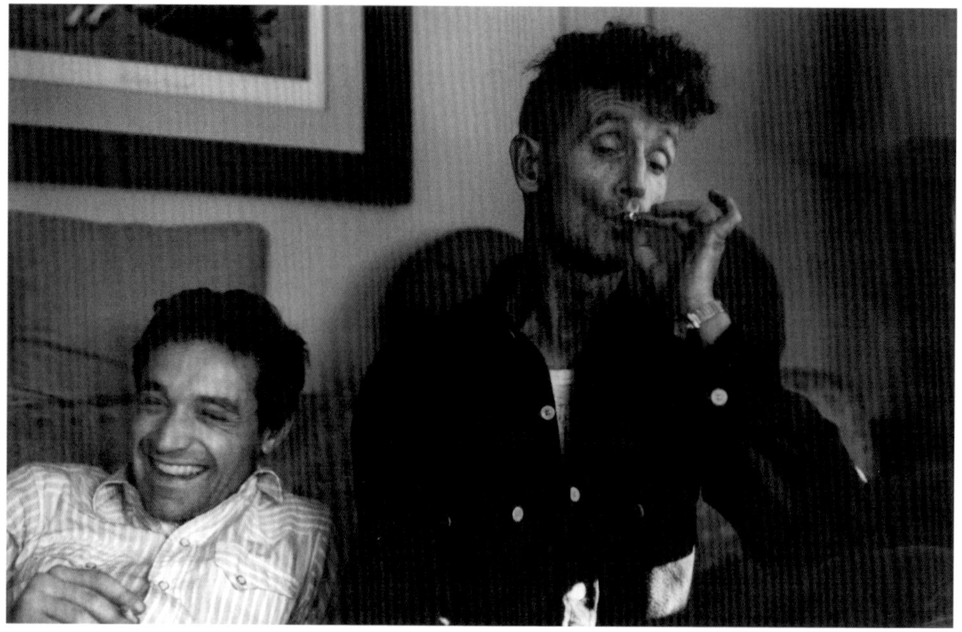

The day after I got off the ship from Europe, a big storm all the way across the Atlantic was blowing hard for the first three days, and I got off that ship and stayed overnight in a hotel in Manhattan, and took a bus the next day out to Greystone Park to see Woody and visited him for about an hour. I can't imagine that I would have stayed more than an hour or two. . . it was marvelous to see how he still was tryin' like hell to stand up straight and walk a straight line—even though he looked like he was drunk or very much fucked up from the disease. Woody was in such a pathetic state, it was very hard to look at him without bustin' out cryin' and it was heartrending just to be in his company. But he always

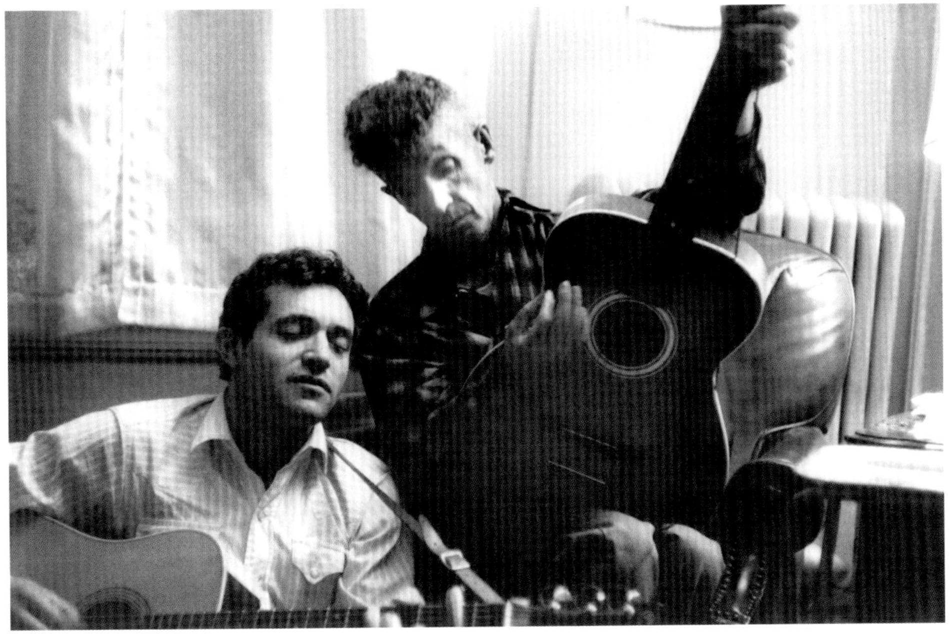

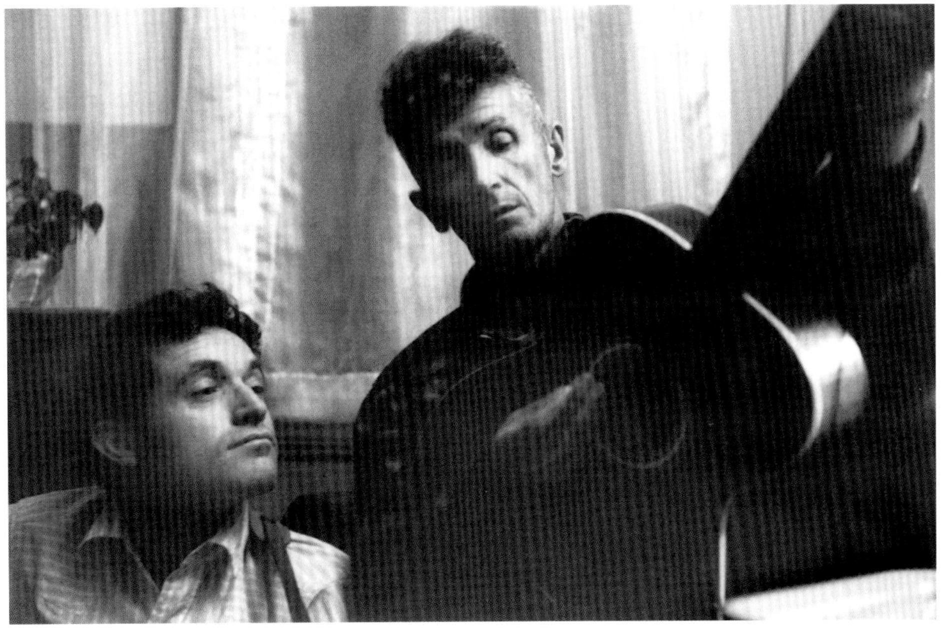

tried to let you know he was still on top of it. He was still in the saddle. He was aware of everything that people were doin' and sayin' and he appreciated it. . . And Bob Dylan was there, a young kid from Minnesota, and we took a bus over to visit the Gleasons, over there in East Orange.

It was nice to see everybody, the friends and admirers, you know. Peter LaFarge was there, and Bob Dylan, and maybe Dave Van Ronk, and I think Maria Muldaur. There might be anywhere from 3 to 6 people at a time on any one given day. It was usually on a Sunday, and Sid cooked chili and beans and corn bread and all of Woody's favorite country cookin'.–*Ramblin' Jack Elliott*

Sometimes we'd bring him in, and he'd have 20 or 30 letters tucked inside of his socks. And then, inside of his shirt and stuck into his pants, he'd have more mail there. He got all this mail. And the first thing we did was to get him in the bathtub. And then Oscar Brand always saw to it that he got a blue shirt and blue jeans instead of you know, dress pants. The ones the hospital had on him, if he'd put his legs in them, he'd disappear. He wasn't a big man, he was small. They gave him clothes, but by gosh, he'd probably wear about a size shirt that you'd put on an 8 or 9-year old kid.–*Sidsel Gleason*

Right: Woody's hospital tee shirt.

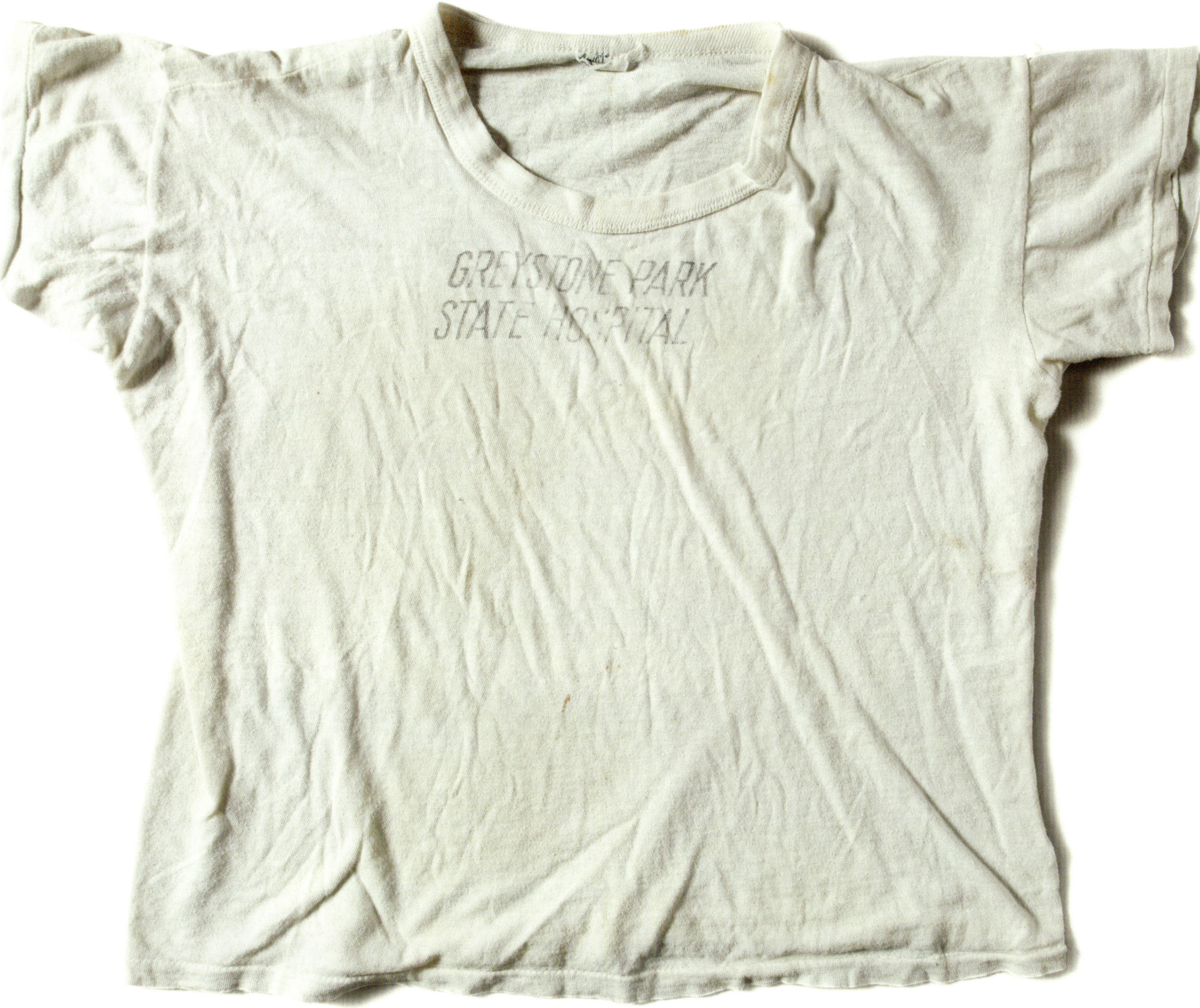
GREYSTONE PARK
STATE HOSPITAL

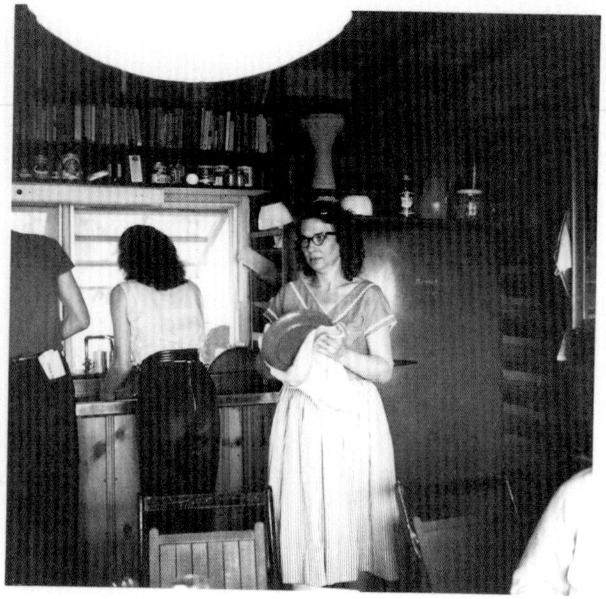

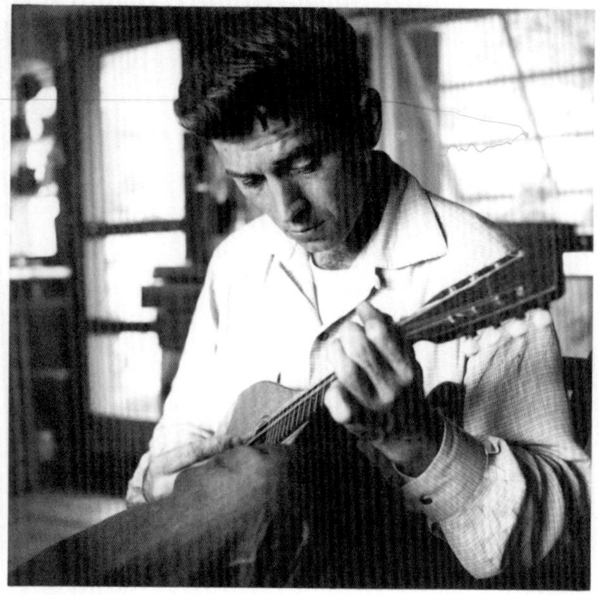

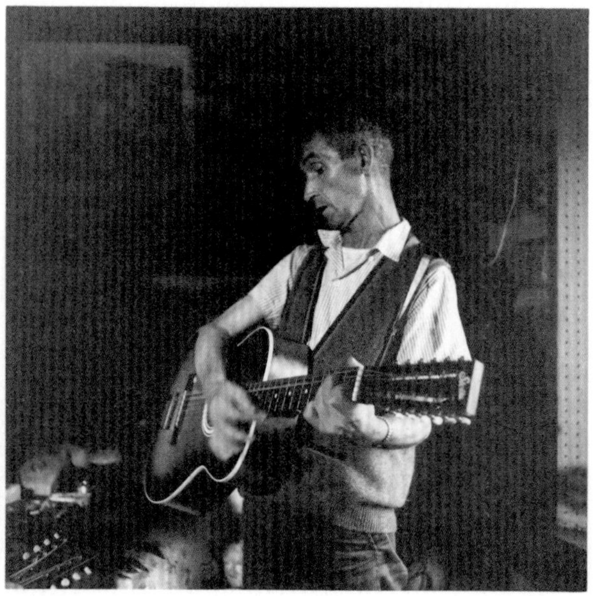

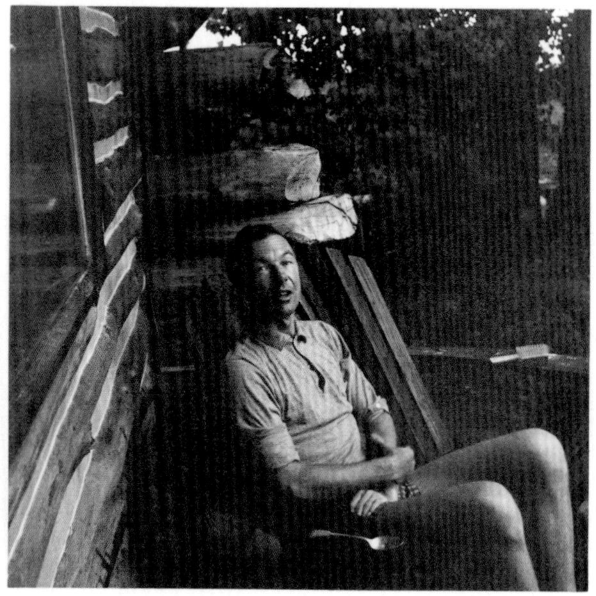

Clockwise: Toshi Seeger and Sidsel Gleason; Ernie Marrs; Pete Seeger; and Woody at the Seeger's home. 1961.

The word got around. Next thing you know, sometimes there'd be 20 or 30 guys or girls who came there. Then they got started playing. And oh man, I tell you we were on the third floor of this apartment. Did you ever hear of washtub bass? Well, there was one of the guys that played washtub bass, and between that and the guitar, it was a pretty wild affair. The people down on the first floor were just about crazy, 'cause it made such a funny noise downstairs. People came from all over, honey, I'm not kidding. They'd come all the way from Oregon. But it was as I said, pretty wild.

There were a lot of them that came. Cisco Houston. . . Jack came back from Europe. And then the other one. . . Peter LaFarge. He was on the cowboy end, too.

(Ramblin' Jack Elliot) would draw Woody sitting on the sofa. . . And Woody sketched some himself. But Woody's weren't very good, honey. They got so where they weren't good because he was ill.

(Bob Dylan would) come out quite often. And sometimes he'd spend a week with us. He was sitting at our kitchen table when he wrote it down (*Song to Woody*). He was always playing Woody's songs, but this was one he wrote.–*Sidsel Gleason*

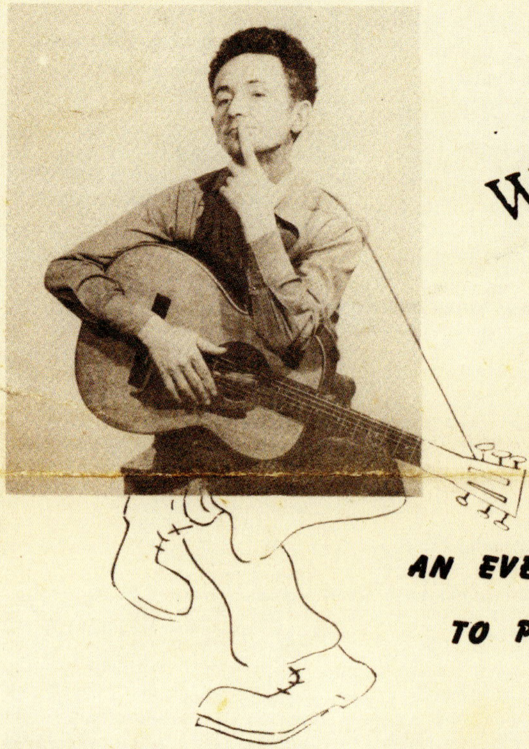

WHERE CAN I GET THAT SONG?

AN EVER-GROWING CATALOGUE AVAILABLE TO PEOPLE'S SONGS MEMBERS ONLY

FOLK

- Acres of Clams (I, 9*)
- Ain't It a Shame (II, 6 and 7)
- All The Pretty Little Horses (III, 6 and 7)
- Big Rock Candy Mountain, The (III, 6 and 7)
- Bonnie Laboring Boy, The (II, 1 and 2)
- Breakdowns and Squares (III, 6 and 7)
- Buffalo Skinners, The (III, 5)
- Caller Herrin' (II, 6 and 7)
- Cold Water (II, 6 and 7)
- Come All Ye Faithful (II, 11)
- Deck the Halls (II, 11)
- Didn't My Lord Deliver, Daniel (III, 4)
- Dodger Song, The (I, 7*)
- Drinking Gourd, The (I, 12)
- Eating Goober Peas (III, 1 and 2)
- Elanoy (III, 6 and 7)
- Farmer is the Man, The (II, 6 and 7)
- Farmer's Curst Wife, The (II, 4)
- Fireship, The (III, 1 and 2)
- First Noel, The (II, 11)
- Four Maries, The (III, 6 and 7)
- Frozen Logger, The (III, 5)
- Go Tell Aunt Nancy (II, 11)
- Go Tell It To the Mountains (II, 11)
- Go Where I send Thee (I, 11)
- God Rest You Merry Gentlemen (II, 11)
- Great Day! (III, 1 and 2)
- Green Sleeves (III, 4)
- Hoosen Johnny (II, 1 and 2)
- I am a Girl of Constant Sorrow (I, 3)
- I Walk the Road Again (I, 3)
- I'm a-Rollin' (II, 10)
- In The Town (II, 11)
- Irene (II, 6 and 7)
- It Takes a Worried Man (II, 3)
- Jenny Jenkins (II, 6 and 7)
- Jingle Bells (II, 11)
- John Hardy (III, 4)
- John Henry (I, 10)
- Joy To the World (II, 11)
- Kevin Barry (II, 5)
- Leave Her, Johnny (II, 5)
- Little Phoebe (II, 1 and 2)
- Little Town of Bethlehem (II, 11)
- Little Willie (II, 1 and 2)
- Midnight Special, The (II, 8)
- Miller Song, The (I, 10)
- My Love is Like a Red, Red Rose (II, 10)
- No Irish Need Apply (III, 4)
- Oh, Freedom (II, 8)
- Original Talking Blues (III, 4)
- Poor Man's Family, The (III, 6 and 7)
- Praties They Grow Small, The (III, 6 and 7)
- Quantrell Side, The (III, 3)
- Runnin', Runnin' (III, 1 and 2)
- Rye Whiskey (II, 6 and 7)
- Silent Night (II, 11)
- Shh, Ta-Ra-Day-Day (II, 5)
- Shorty George (III, 3)
- Scots Wha' Ha'e (III, 4)
- Slavery's Chain (III, 1 and 2)
- So Long, It's Been Good to Know You (II, 5)
- State Of Arkansas (III, 1 and 2)
- Stir the Puddin' (II, 3)
- Tom Dooley (III, 1 and 2)
- Three Kings, The (II, 11)
- Twelve Days Of Christmas (II, 11)
- We Wish You a Merry Christmas (II, 11)

UNION

- Casey Jones (I, 1)
- Eight Hours (III, 1)
- Eight Hour Day (II, 3)
- Get Thee Behind Me, Satan (II, 4)
- Great Day! (II, 1 and 2)
- Horse With a Union Label (II, 4)
- Hold The Fort (II, 3)
- I Went Down To The Steel Mill (I, 2*)
- I'm The Guy (I, 2*)
- I've Got a Date on a Picket Line (I, 2*)
- Joe Hill (II, 8)
- Keep That Line A-Moving (I, 2*)
- May Day Song (I, 3)
- Miner's Lifeguard (I, 12)
- My Union Man (II, 10)
- Newspapermen (I, 10)
- Picketline Priscilla (I, 6*)
- Poor Old C. E. Wilson (I, 2*)
- Roll The Union On (I, 1)
- Roll Out The Union (II, 3)
- Scabs Crawl In,The (I, 2*)
- Selling Union (III, 1 and 2)
- Solidarity Forever (I, 1)
- Talking Union (I, 9*)
- Taft-Hartley Blues (II, 9)
- "T" Stands For Tobacco (II,6 and 7)
- Teacher's Blues (II, 3)
- U. A. W.-C. I. O. (II, 8)
- Union Man, The (II, 1 and 2)
- Union Maid (I, 7*)
- Union Gang (I, 5)
- Union Square Dance (I, 3)
- Union Way, The (I, 10)
- Unity Rhumba (II, 6 and 7)
- We Are Building a Strong Union (III, 3)
- We Are The Guys (II,1 and 2)
- We'll Picket Once And Picket Twice (I, 2*)
- We Pity Our Bosses Five (I, 1)
- We Shall Not Be Moved (II, 3)
- Which Side Are You On? (II, 1 and 2)
- Winnsboro Cotton Mill Blues (I, 8)
- Whole Wide World Around, The (II, 6 and 7)
- You Gotta Go Down (I, 3)
- You Guys Gotta Organize (I, 7*)

CHILDREN

- All Work Together (II, 3)
- All the Pretty Little Horses (III, 6 and 7)
- Bear Story, A (I, 3)
- Bling! Blang! (II, 8)
- Brown Skinned Cow (II, 11)
- Children, Go Where I Send Thee (I, 11)
- Don't You Push Me (II, 6 and 7)
- Everything Is Higher (II, 6 and 7)
- Go Tell Aunt Nancy (II, 11)
- Riding the Dragon (II, 5)
- Shh Ta-Ra-Dah-Day (II, 5)
- When I was a Little Boy (I, 6*)

People's Songs is a non-profit →

- 1 -

Left: "People's Songs" magazine.
Below: Bob Dylan, New York. 1962.
Right: Lyrics to "Song to Woody" handwritten by Bob Dylan.

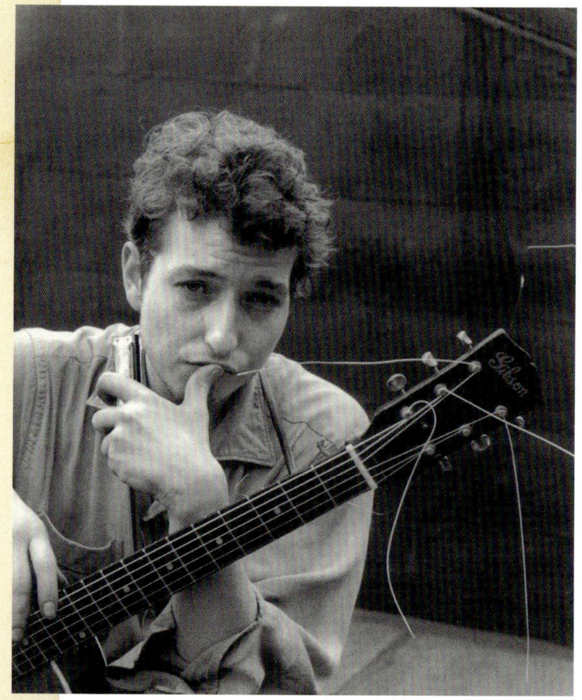

1. I'm out here a thousand miles from my home
walkin the road other men gone down
I'm seeing your people, your places ~~and~~ things
Your paupers and princes and peasants and kings

2. Hey Woody I wrote you a song
~~Bout~~ Bout this funny old world that's coming along
It's sick and it's hungry, it's tired and torn
Almost dead and it ain't even born

3. Hey Woody Guthrie, I know that you know
The things that I'm saying and many times more
I'm singing this song but I can't sing enough
Cause there's not many men done the things that you done

4. Here's to Cisco and Sonny and Leadbelly too
And all the good people that traveled with you
Here's to the hands and the hearts of the men
That come with the dust and are gone with the wind

5. I'm leaving tommorow, I could leave today
But way down on that road somewhere
The very last thing that I want to do
~~Is~~ is to say I been hitting some hard traveling too.

Written by Bob Dylan
In Mills Bar on Bleeker St in
New York City on 14th day of February
for
Woody Guthrie

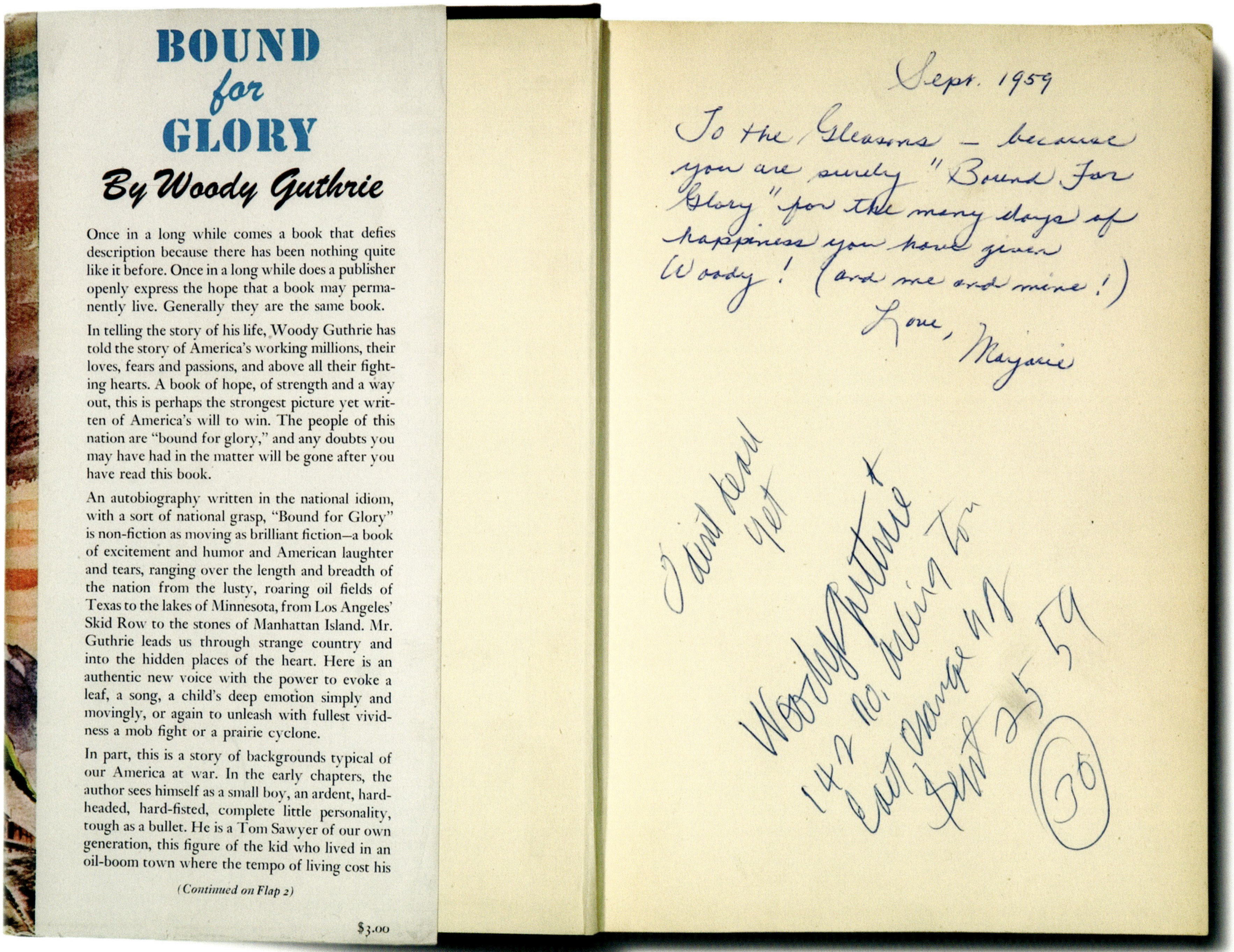

"Bound For Glory," signed by Woody and Marjorie for the Gleasons.

I'm telling you, that was the wildest time. All those people would come in there, and I wouldn't have any idea about some of them, and all of a sudden here people would be coming from different places, and it was wild. It was really something. And my husband, he loved music, and he'd sit there and he'd pat his foot to keep time with the music. Oh honey, it was wild, it was wild. Sometimes I wondered, would it ever quit? 'Cause people would come from miles and miles and miles when they found out that he was there. And the parties we had! And that was when I made the cowboy stew, my gosh there was so many of them come. Oscar (Brand) was the one who gave me the money to get the food because we just couldn't afford it to feed everybody.–*Sidsel Gleason*

One time I'd taken Woody from one of the concerts in New York, at Cooper Union, and we were driving him back to Greystone. I remember we were sitting in the front of the Greystone main building, and we'd been talking about this and that. The Ramblers were working on a brochure—I think Woody had seen us play that day, and he liked us playing the old time music and all, so we said, "Hey, Woody, would you give us some kind of a quote that we could use about us?" And he said, "Oh yeah, New Lost City Ramblers are the best—after me." And we used it. It was really funny, you know. I felt a little guilty about asking him to do it, but he was very folkie and funny.*—John Cohen*

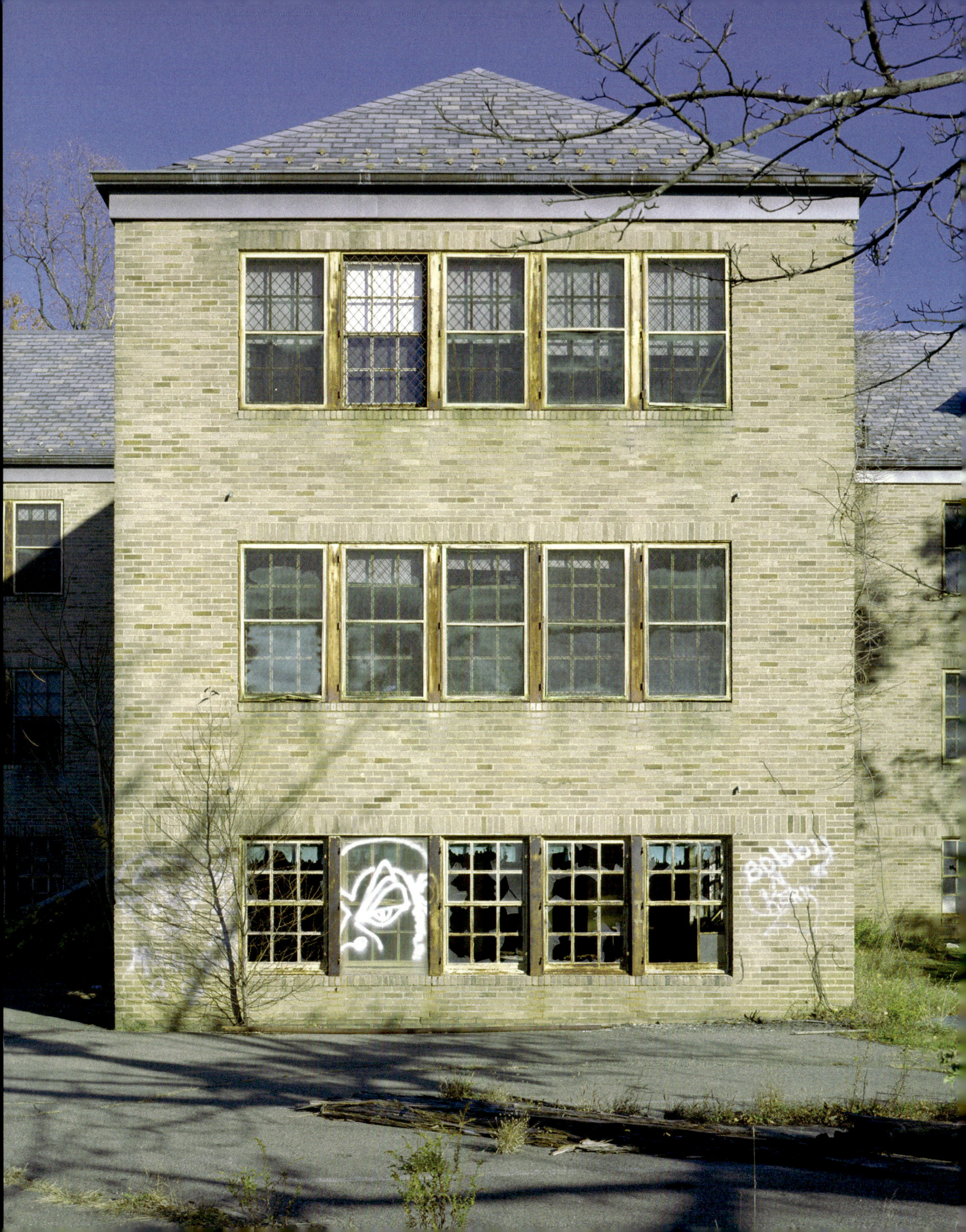

At some point, my mother realized that it would be even better to bring my father home on Sundays, rather than visit him at the hospital. At least we kids would be able to stay around the house, able to enjoy our day off. So she would drive the hour and a half to Greystone, pick him up, bring him home, spend the day and drive him back in the evening. All in all it was a three-hour drive. At that time, they had not yet finished the Verrazano Bridge, which would cut off about forty-five minutes from the trip. It's funny, to this day, whenever I see this great expansive bridge, all I can think about is how relieved and happy my mother would have been if it had been completed while my father was still at Greystone.–*Nora Guthrie*

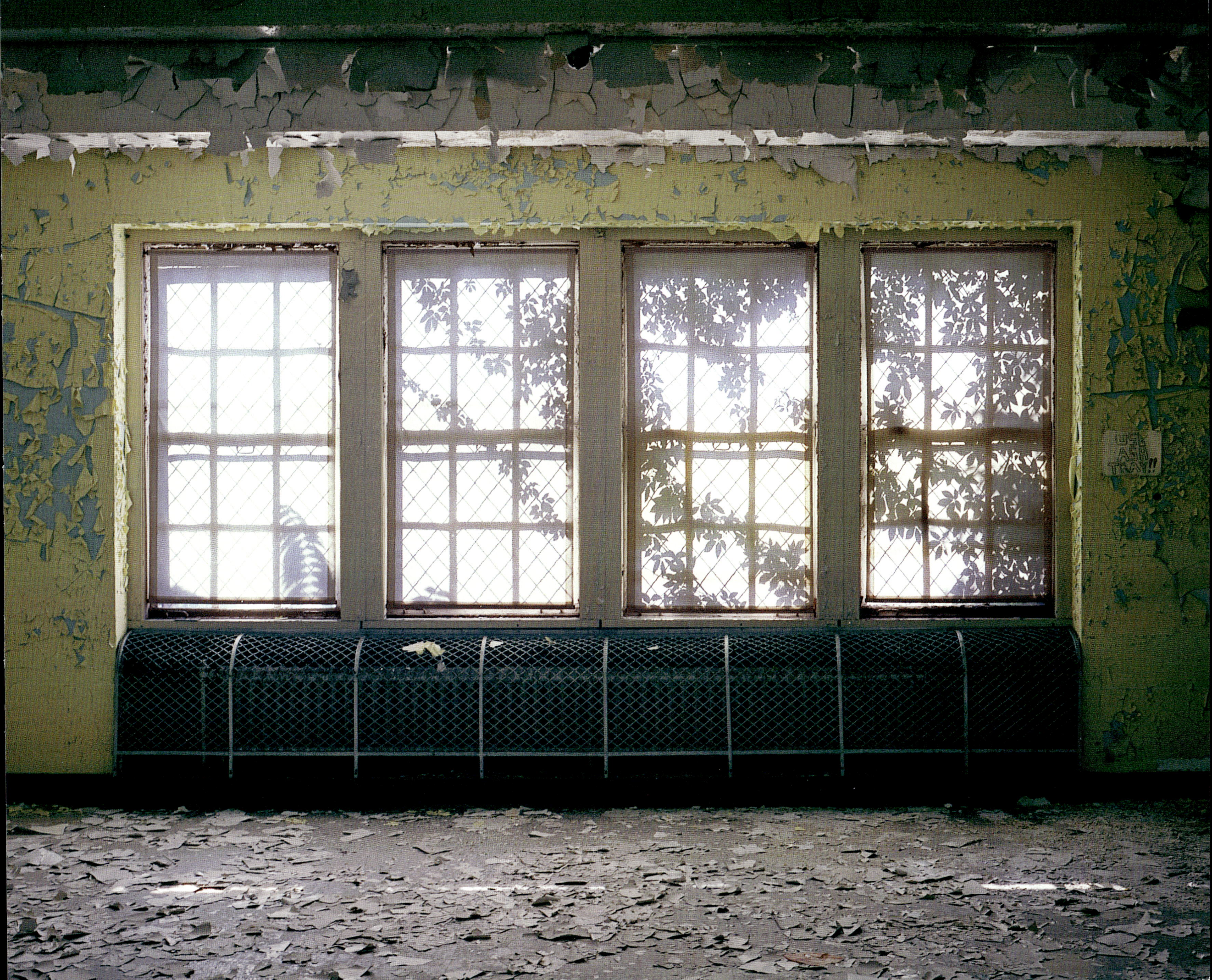
USE ASH TRAY!!

There were other occasions where I had picked him up, or I had somebody pick him up for me. We had various events with the Weavers. I'd want him to be there, and we'd pick him up for the day, bring him here, and usually Marjorie would take him back.–*Harold Leventhal*

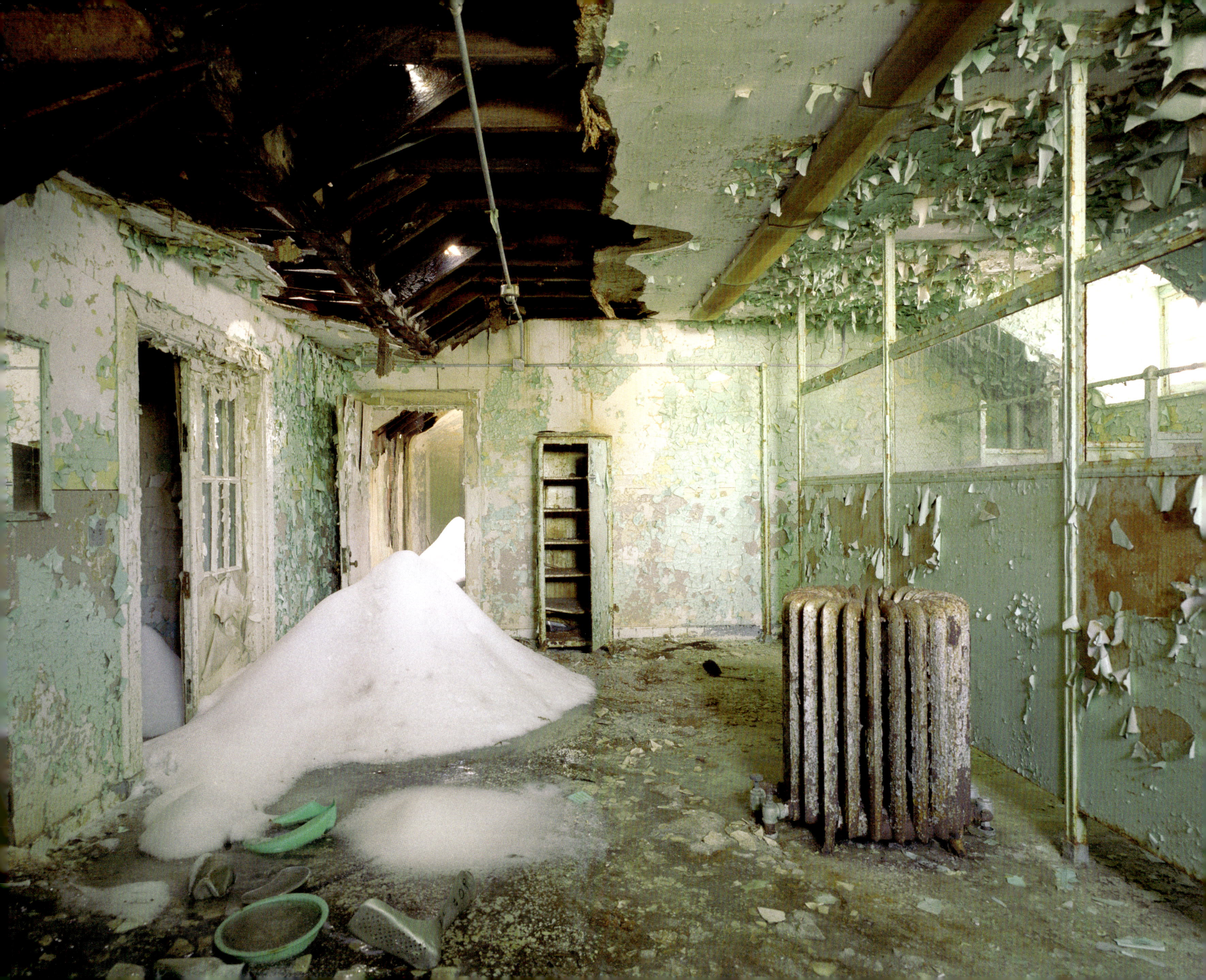

Alan Lomax had this big program at Carnegie Hall. It was called "Folksongs '59," and I'd been photographing it, but I was with Woody, and we were sitting up in a box on the left hand side of the stage at Carnegie Hall. I remember being very moved by the fact that Pete was on stage and he sang—I think he acknowledged that Woody was there—and then he sang that beautiful song, "Deportees," that I knew that Woody had only done as a poem.

He had never done music to it, and now someone else had put the music to that song, and Woody was sitting next to me reciting it. That's a private thing that I'll share. At the same time, there's this huge hall with Pete up there singing and getting everybody to sing. They had the big public version of it; I'm hearing the private version of it. It was very touching. I just remembered that. Almost indescribable, although I just tried to describe it.—*John Cohen*

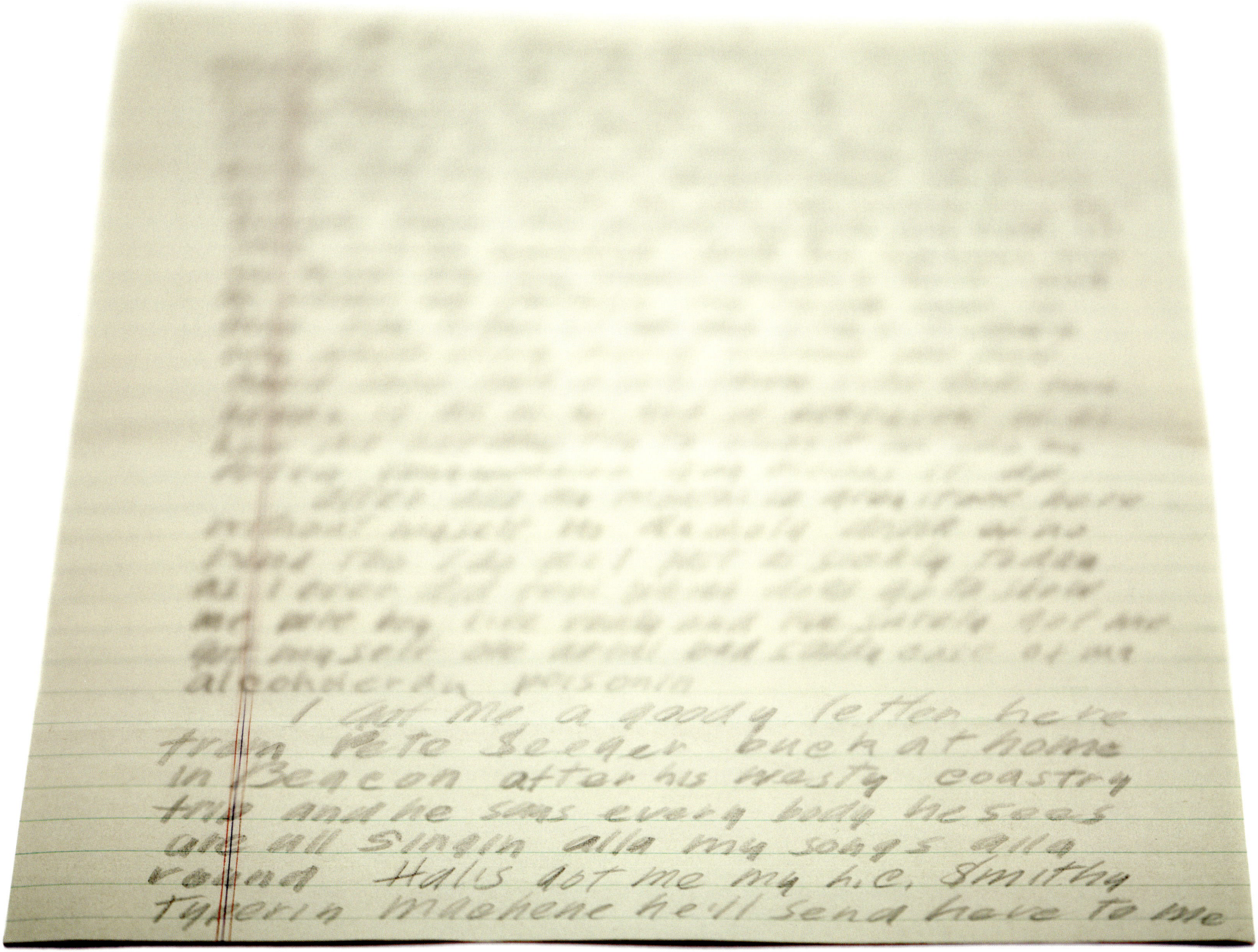
I got me a goody letter here from Pete Seeger back at home in Beacon after his nasty coastry trip and he says every body he sees are all singin alla my songs alla round Hal's got me my h.c. Smithy typerin machene he'll send here to me

"I got me a goody letter here from Pete Seeger ... he says every body he sees are all singin alla my songs alla round." Woody. 1956.

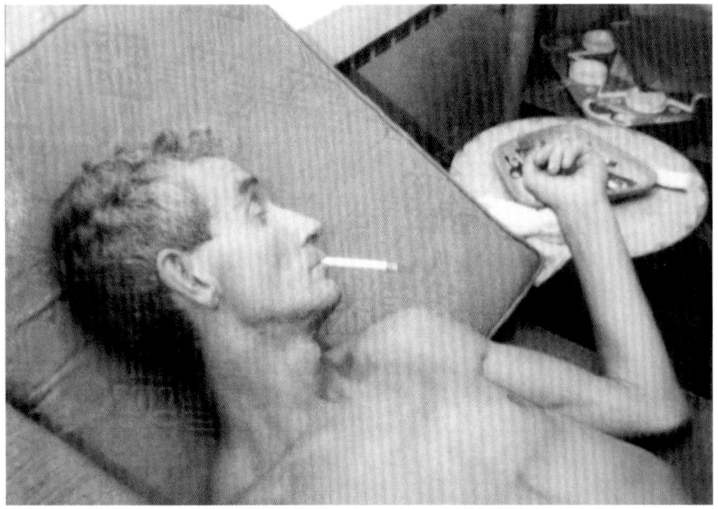

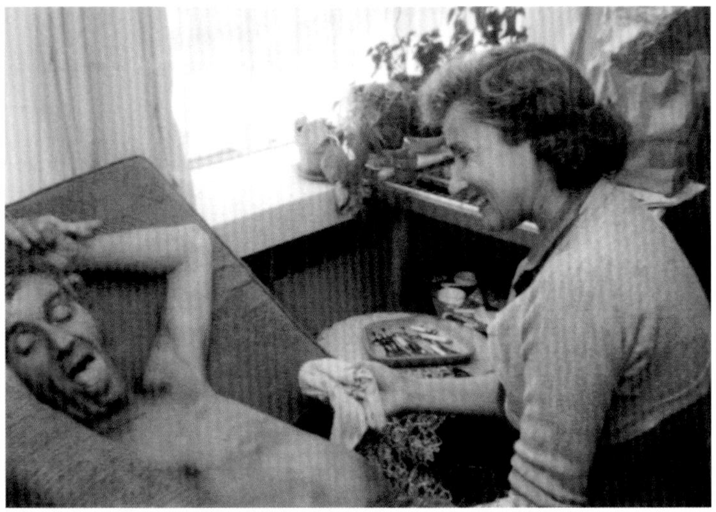

Woody and Marjorie at home. Howard Beach, Queens. 1961.

My father needed so much care. One of the symptoms of Huntington's is the body's constant motion, which burns up a large amount of calories. My mother piled my father with high caloric foods: chocolate cakes and quarts of milk, hot dogs, fried chicken, blocks of honeycomb–anything to put back the pounds that he had lost during the week. She stripped him of his clothes and scrubbed him in the bath, sprinkling him afterwards with talcum powder and singing, "Doesn't he smell sweet now!" She would wash and iron his clothes, sew up the tears, and dress him up like a mother dressing her child for a first day of school. She would sit with him in the living room as he lay on the couch, lighting cigarettes for him, hand-feeding him, holding his arms down while his records played on the record player. She was constantly on call until it was time to head back to Greystone.–*Nora Guthrie*

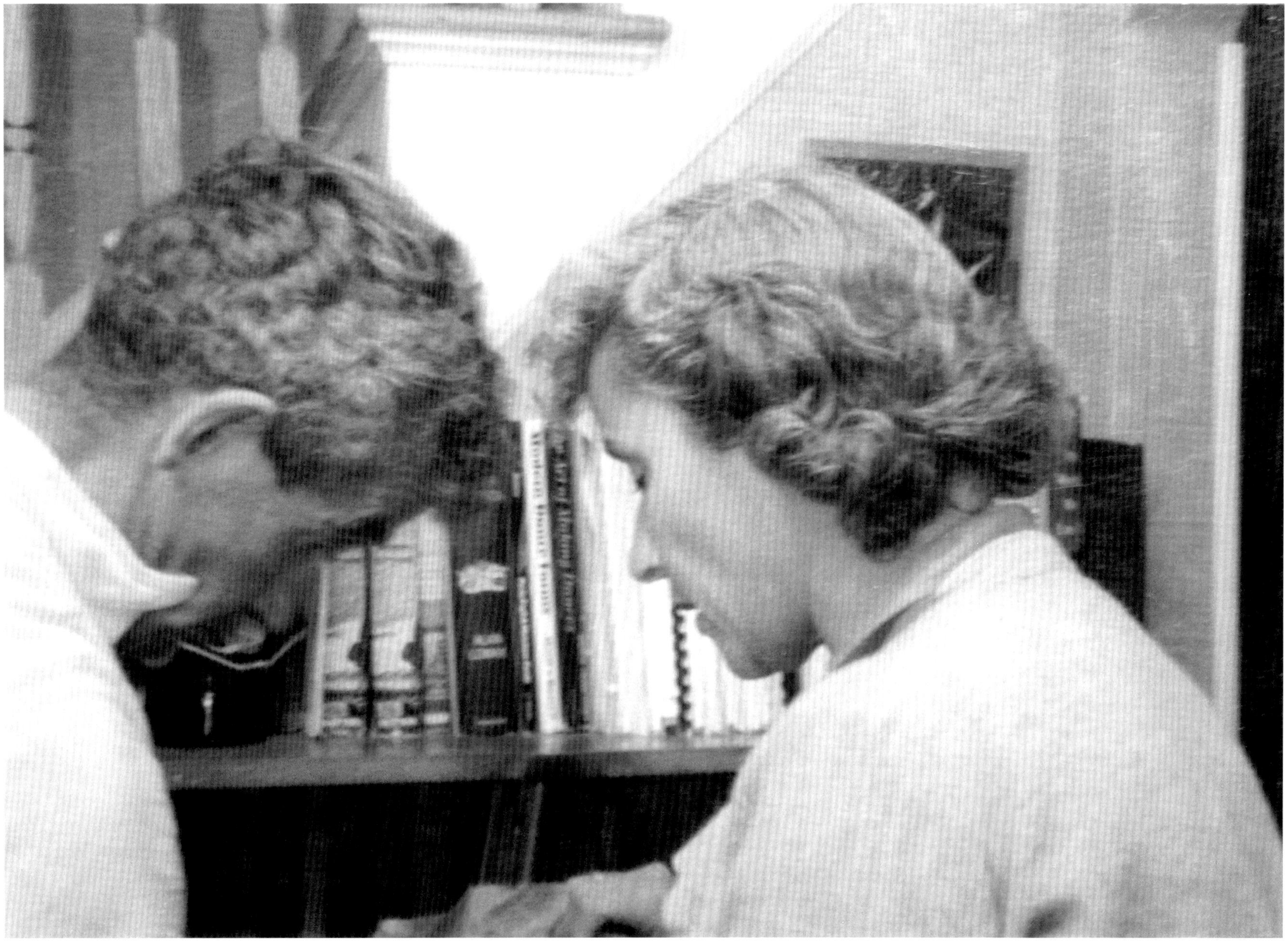

In our family, my mom and dad had an obvious love for each other that extended beyond their marriage, extended before their marriage—through it—and beyond it. A love and appreciation for each other as artists and human beings and as parents. And I think she tried to make the most of that under very difficult circumstances—not to everyone's complete satisfaction, ever. But she did the best she could and I think she thought it was important to maintain some kind of family relationship.

Even though she was married to other people at the time, and even though my dad had been remarried at one point briefly. They had one of those timeless movie-type of loves, you know. And it's very obvious in all of their writing and all of their actions. They would sit together, and they would talk, and they would share their lives as best they could.—*Arlo Guthrie*

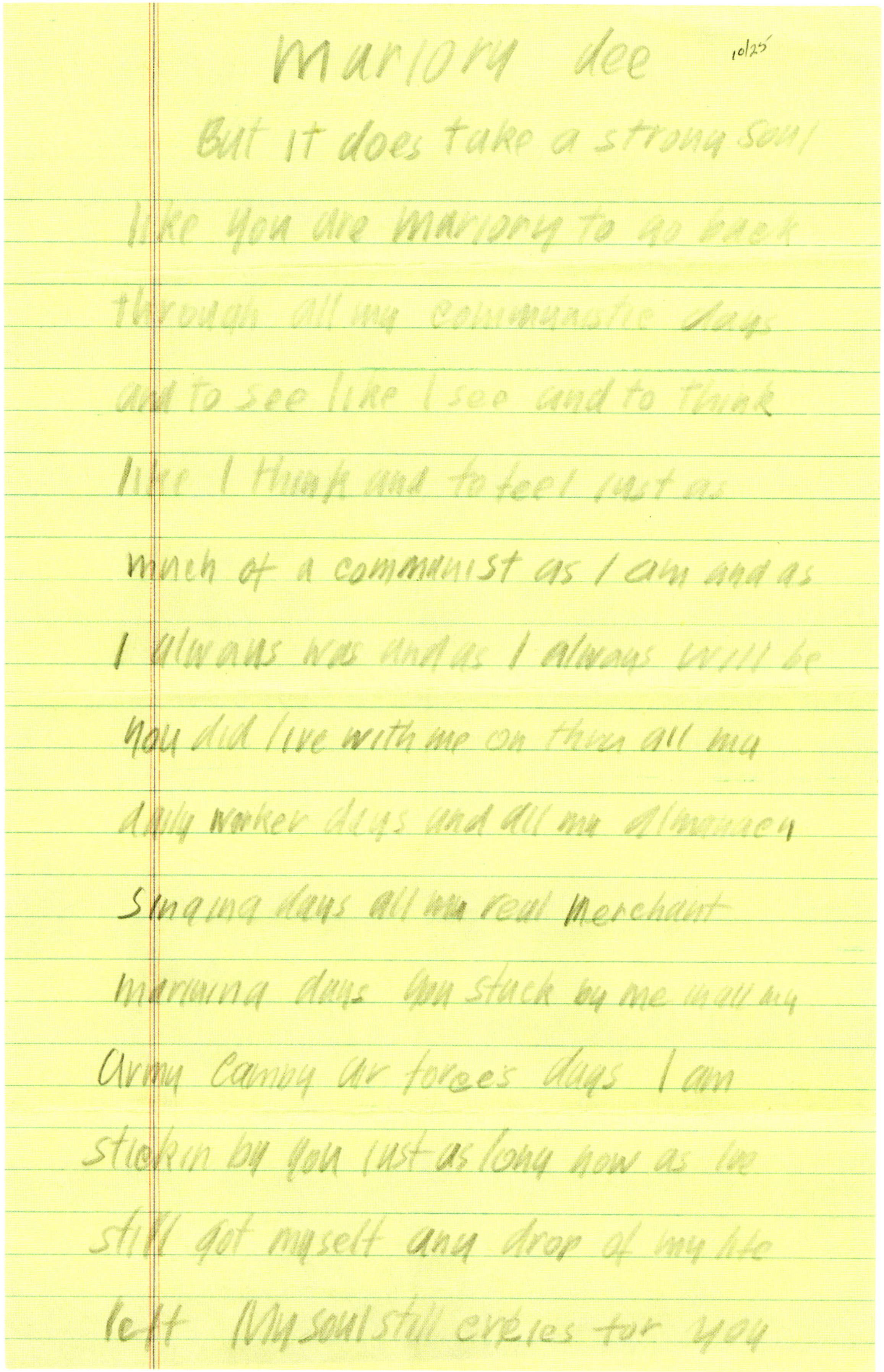

Marjory dee 10/25

But it does take a strong soul
like you are marjory to go back
through all my communistic days
and to see like I see and to think
like I think and to feel just as
much of a communist as I am and as
I always was and as I always will be
you did live with me on thru all my
daily worker days and all my almanac
singing days all my real merchant
marining days you stuck by me in all my
army camp air forces days I am
stickin by you just as long now as Ive
still got myself any drop of my life
left My soul still cries for you

Woody's letter to his wife, Marjorie. October 25, 1956.

I liked him as a patient. He always smiled to me whenever I passed by, or when I took care of him. With me, he was always very, very pleasant. He did not interact too much with staff or with patients, because he had difficulties in articulating words. He was in the late stage of Huntington's Chorea. . . He was walking around a little bit but he walked with some difficulties. . . Generally, there was no change except that sometimes he tended to choke. . . from not being able to swallow well. Huntington's Chorea is characterized by choreo-athetoid movements of the arms and muscular groups, slowly affects all muscular groups impairing the ability to walk, to talk, to swallow, and so on. And on some of these occasions we felt we should take some X-rays to make sure that there was no aspiration, no pneumonitis, or anything like that.

There was no treatment. The only thing that was done at that time was utilizing the side effect of Thorazine. Thorazine tends to give a degree of muscular spasticity that counteracts the choreoid movements of Huntington's. Basically, the patient may have better control of his movement, but the effects are modest. But, of course, it's not a treatment.

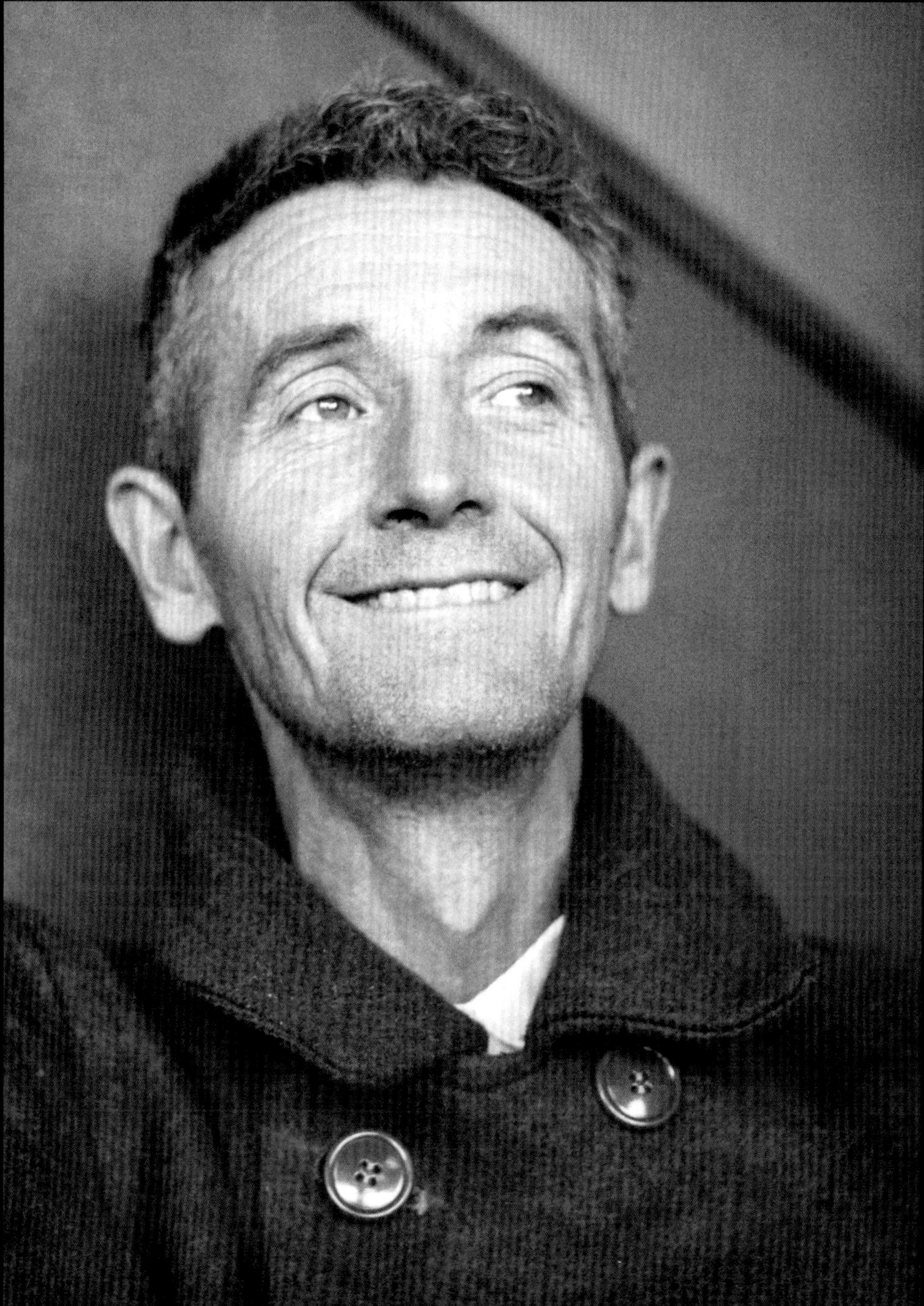

I remember his smile. It was not a big smile.

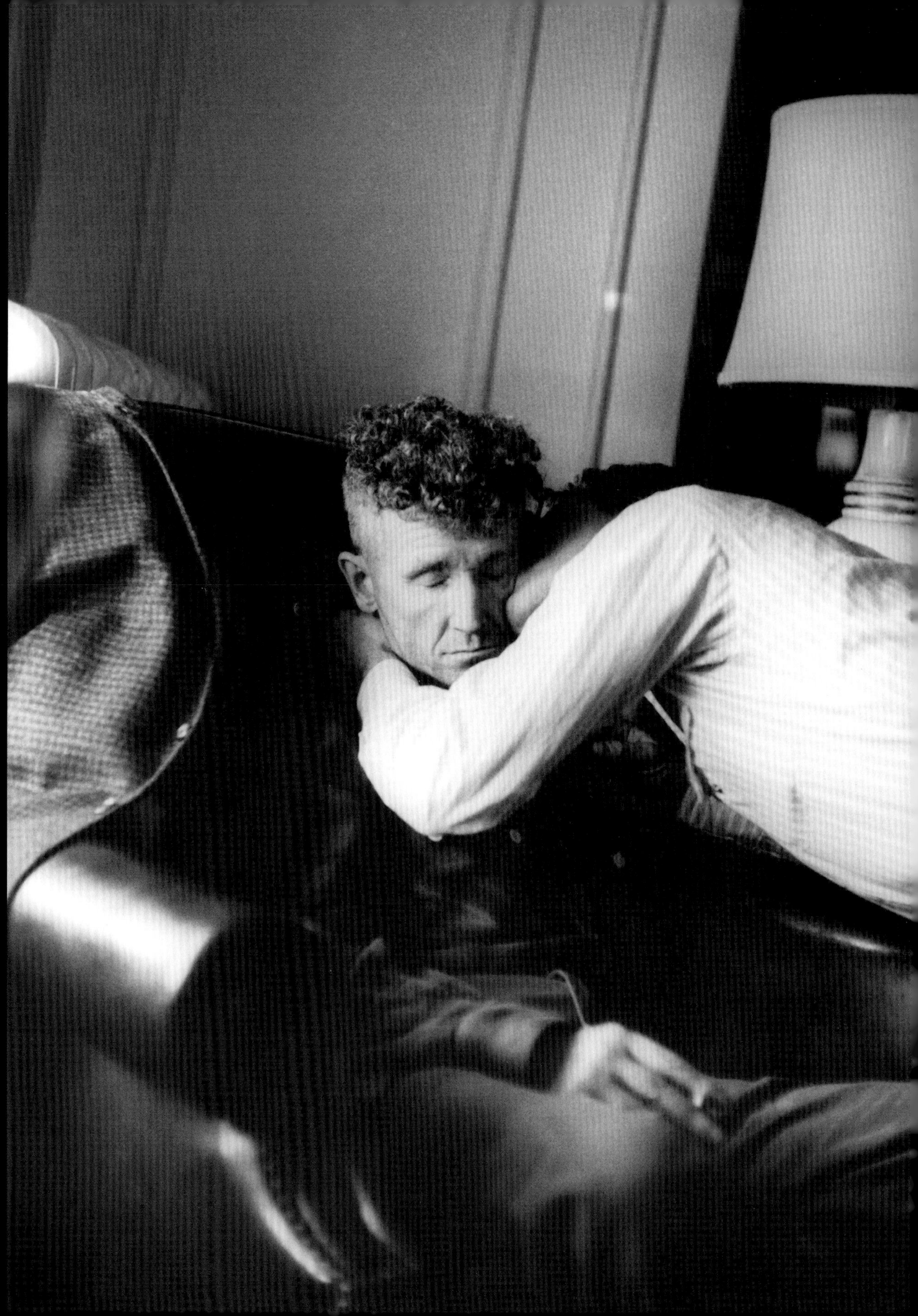

Huntington's is what took his mother away at a very young age, and if you're gonna do "what if," you could say, what if she hadn't had Huntington's? But he had all that other shit happen to him due to his mother being taken away from Huntington's and that was the beginning of a lot of tragedy in his life.

Woody was dogged by tragedy, with his sister who caught up in a fire, and there were a great number of Americans experiencing a lot of tragedy because there was so much hunger and starvation back in those days in the Dust Bowl and the Depression and rich people losing their money in 1929, and jumping off of buildings and stuff.

If he didn't have the Chorea, I think that he might have, maybe, lived to be 90. He was otherwise very rugged, wiry, and his disposition was straight. I think he would have lived longer, perhaps made even a bigger contribution than he did—but I don't see how anybody could possibly make a bigger contribution in the writing world. It's hard to imagine. *–Ramblin' Jack Elliott*

Woody and Ramblin' Jack Elliott. 1960.

Marjorie was very protective of Woody, and Marjorie didn't really want anybody to know how bad it was. She was always underestimating the burden. But it was really tough. Woody was unpredictable, and sometimes it was hard to differentiate between Woody and his illness–because the illness itself led to these movements, but also to a change of personality. Marjorie also spoke of going to the hospital as frequently as she did, and the exhaustion associated with it, and the frustration with the medical system. She spoke of the difficulty getting the care that she wanted for Woody and that he needed, and the lack of knowledge and the impact of the lack of knowledge.–*Dr. Michael Hayden*

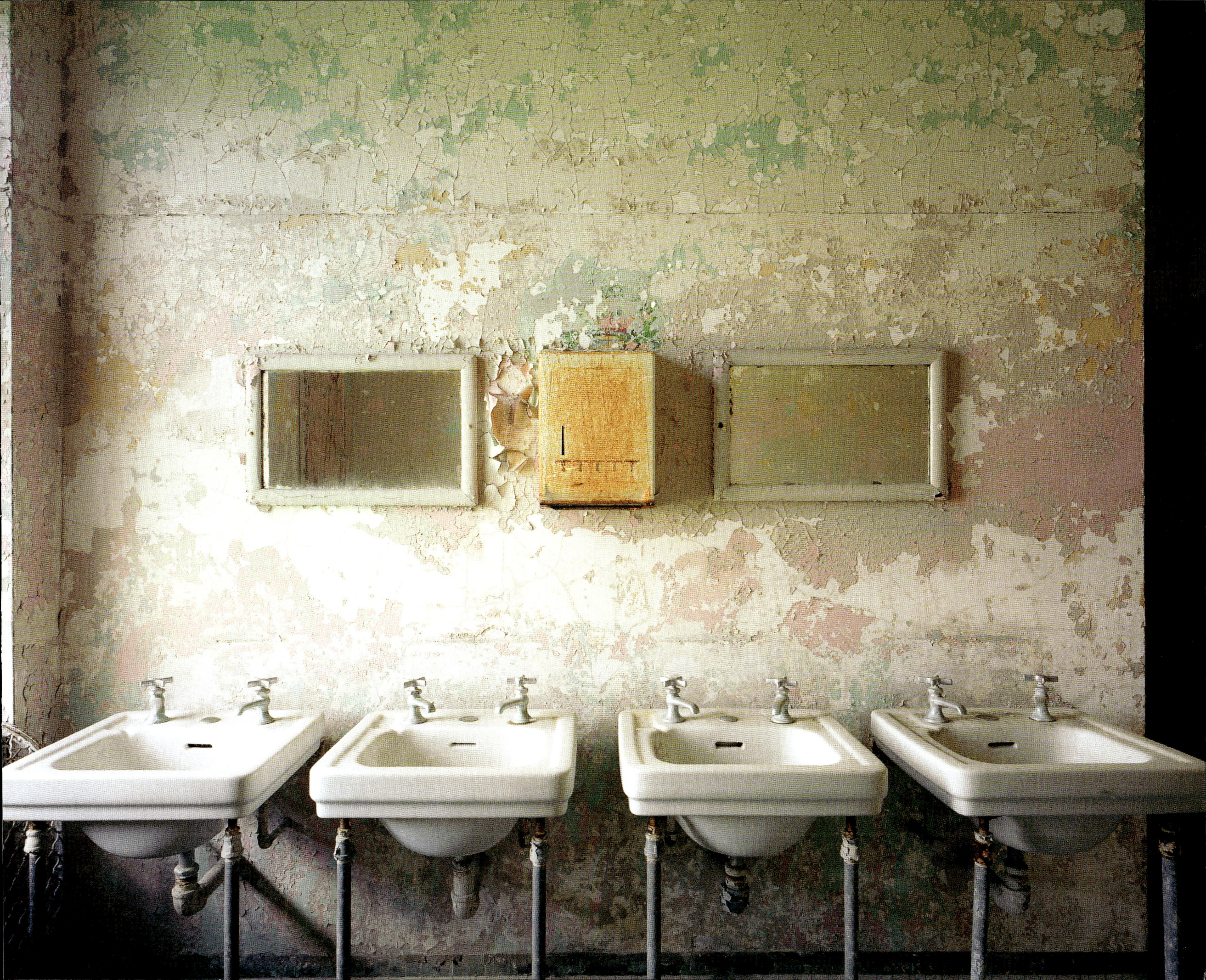

We didn't want people going out because Woody could not talk. People came to look at him. Just friends were allowed. To have other visitors that he didn't know, they would just be looking at him. It would hurt his feelings. I'd come out, and Bing Crosby recorded one of his songs and I'd play it for him. I played "Alice's Restaurant" for him. He was amused by it.–*Harold Leventhal*

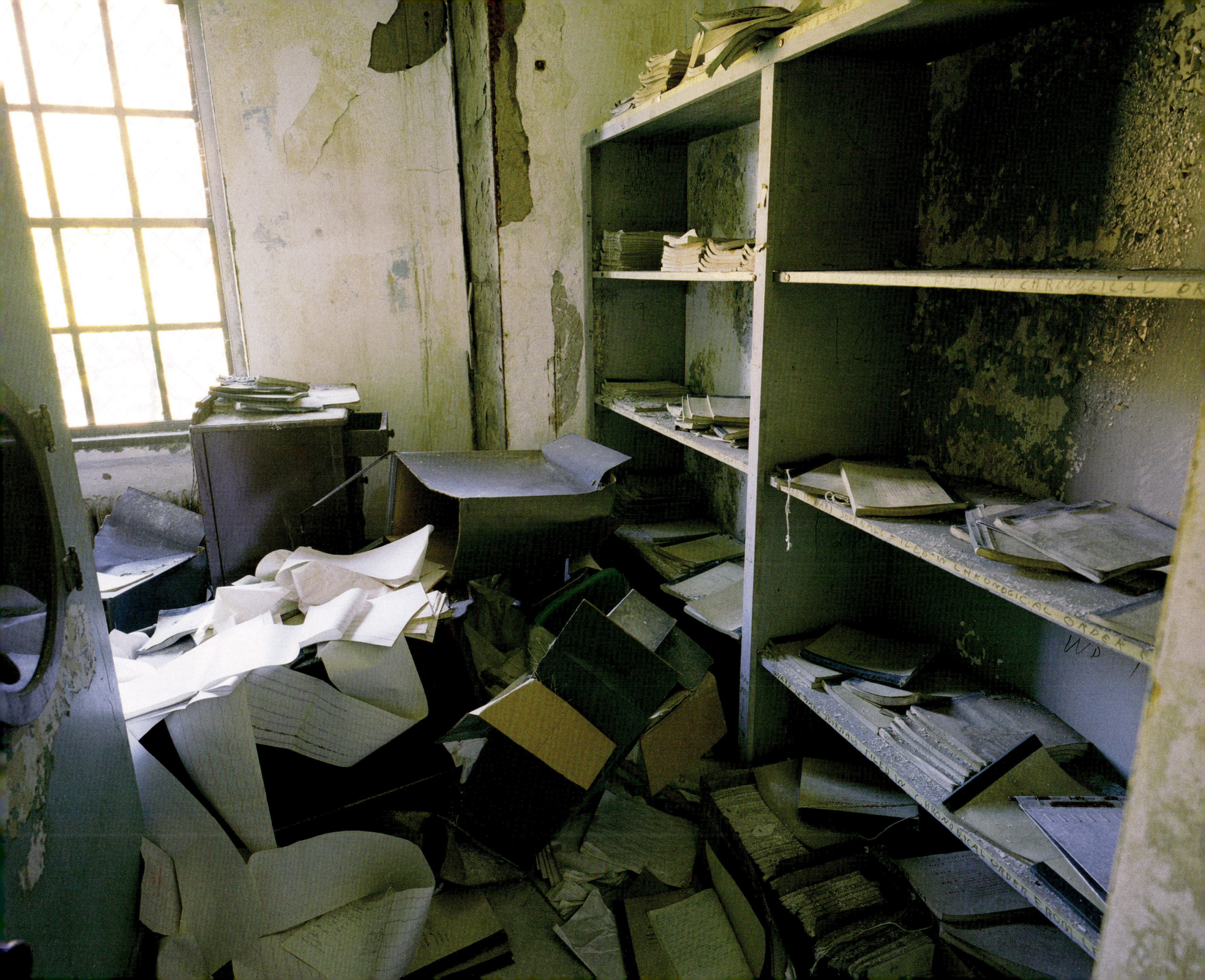

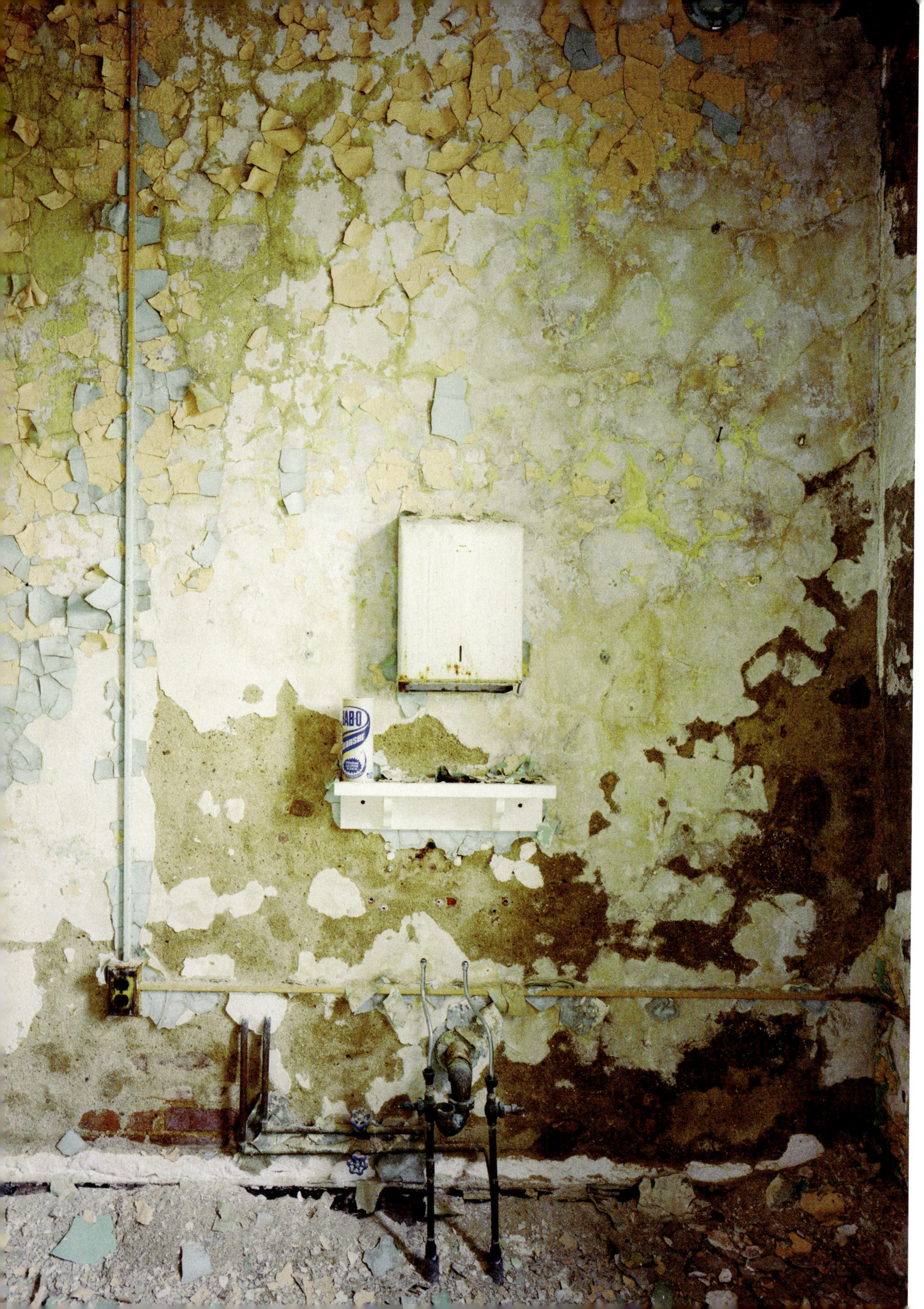

All this time he was trying to write. His beautiful handwriting was deteriorating, but he still wanted me to bring long yellow pads to the hospital. He filled them up with his "scrapples," and I replaced them with additional tablets. He loved the feel of his pencils and tried to keep one always on him. Which wasn't easy in a ward with 40 men, mostly patients with mental disorders.–*Marjorie Guthrie*

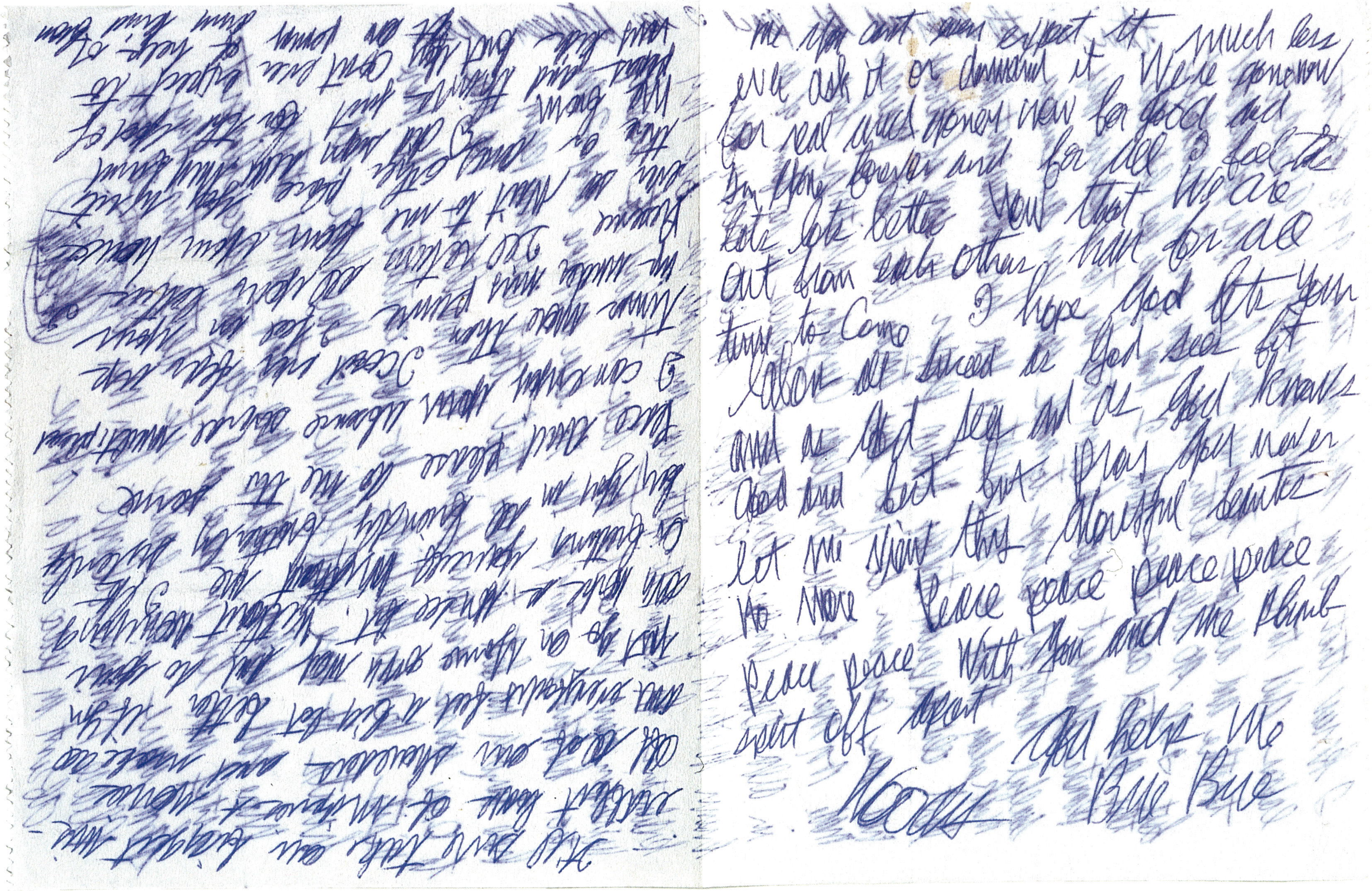

me they can't even expect it much less
ever ask it or demand it We're gonna
for real and honey now for good and
for long forever and for all I feel
lots lots better now that we are
out from each other here for all
time to come I hope God lets you
alone all sweet as God sees fit
and as they say and as God knows
good and best but pray you never
let me view this [illegible]
no more Peace peace peace peace
peace peace with you and me plumb
spirit off apart
You help me
Woody
Bye Bye

Woody's letter to his wife, Marjorie, written on paper towels. December 1956.

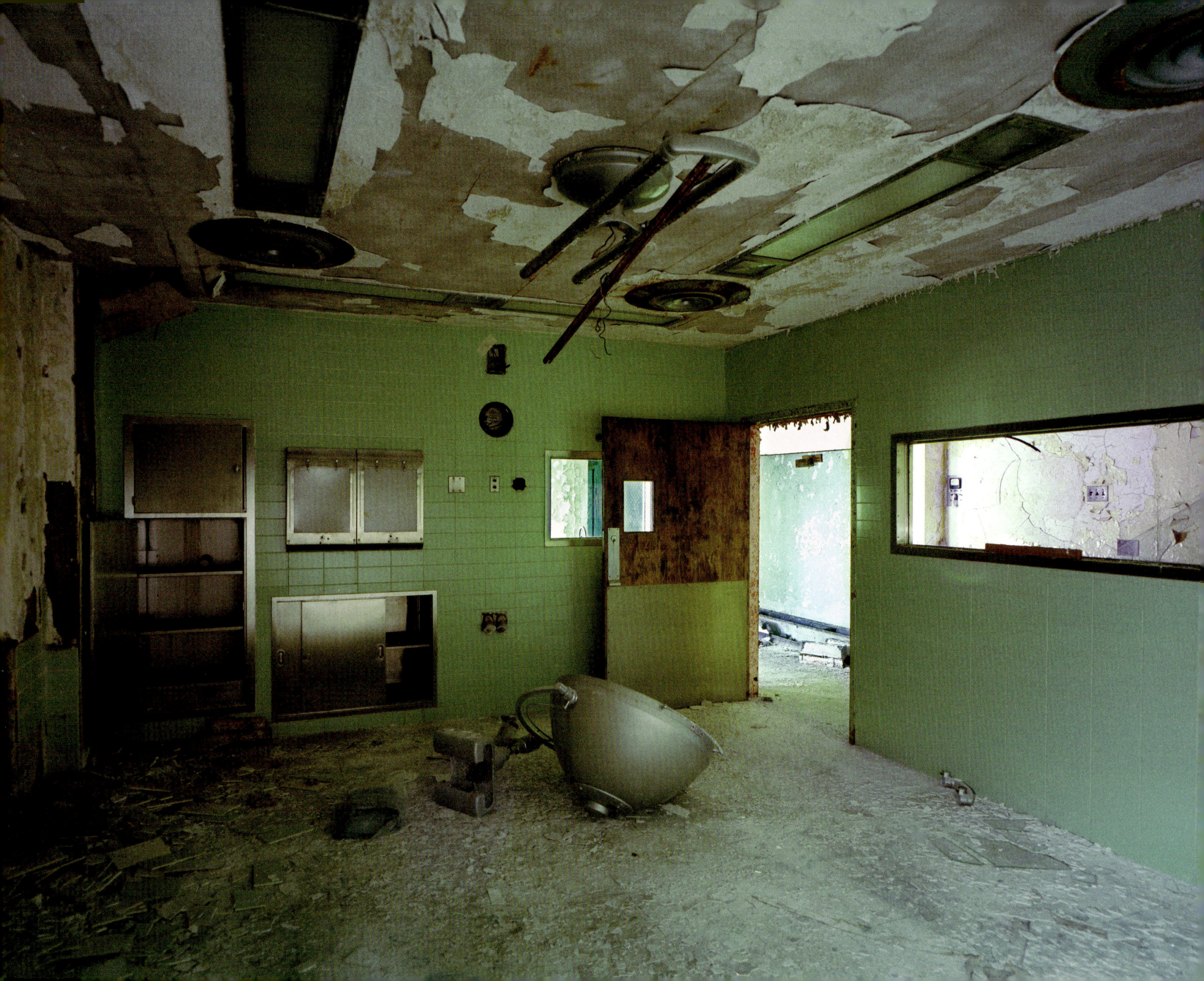

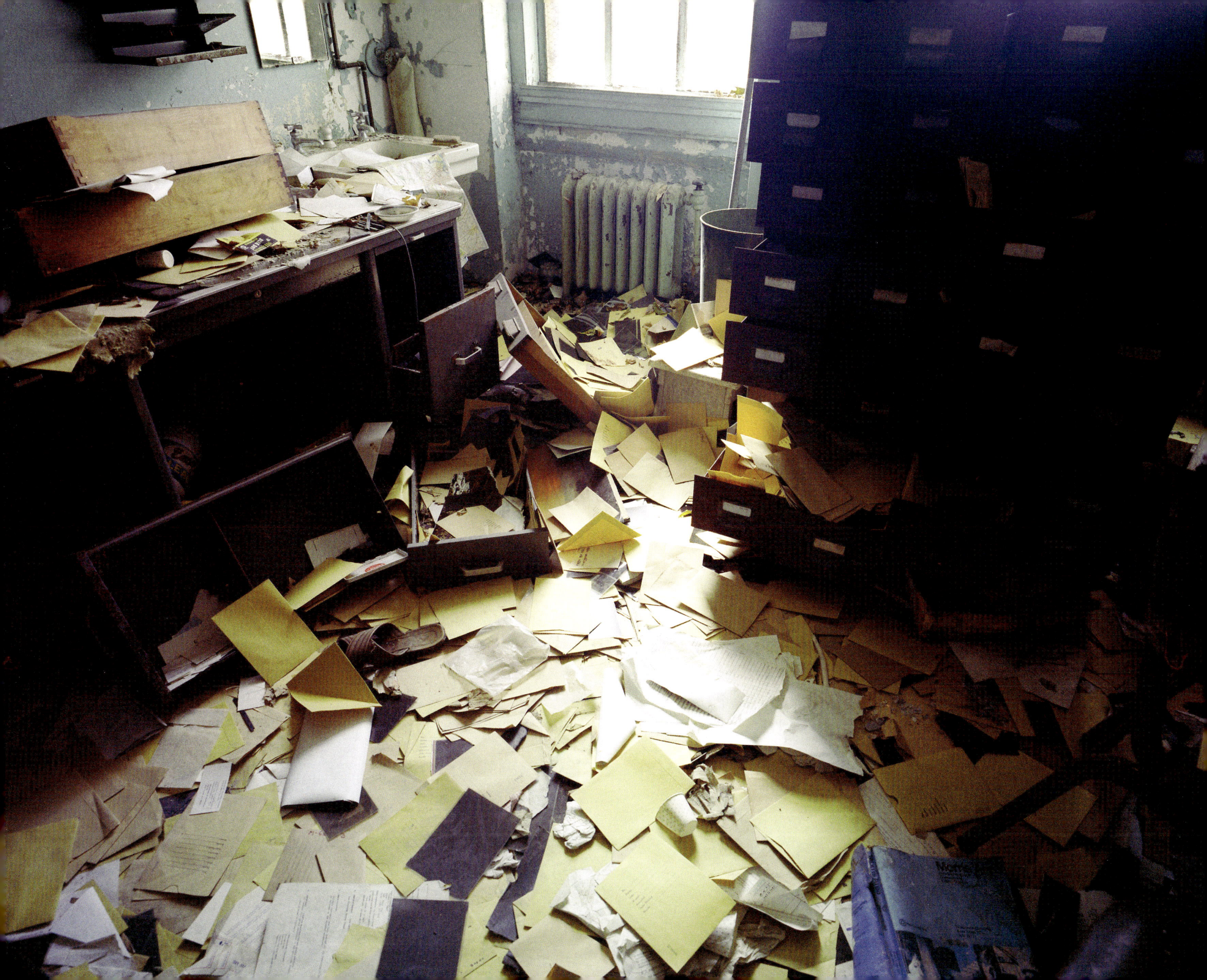

more give ... days

album, a few

n Hi fi machene and the

ng enough to write down my

~~#~~ christe ballad and the

realy still believe or was it

mood of some moment and

lieve more in god more (and in Jesus)

minute that passe

I aint dead quite yet

Woody Guthrie

Woody fatty lady 195

(30)

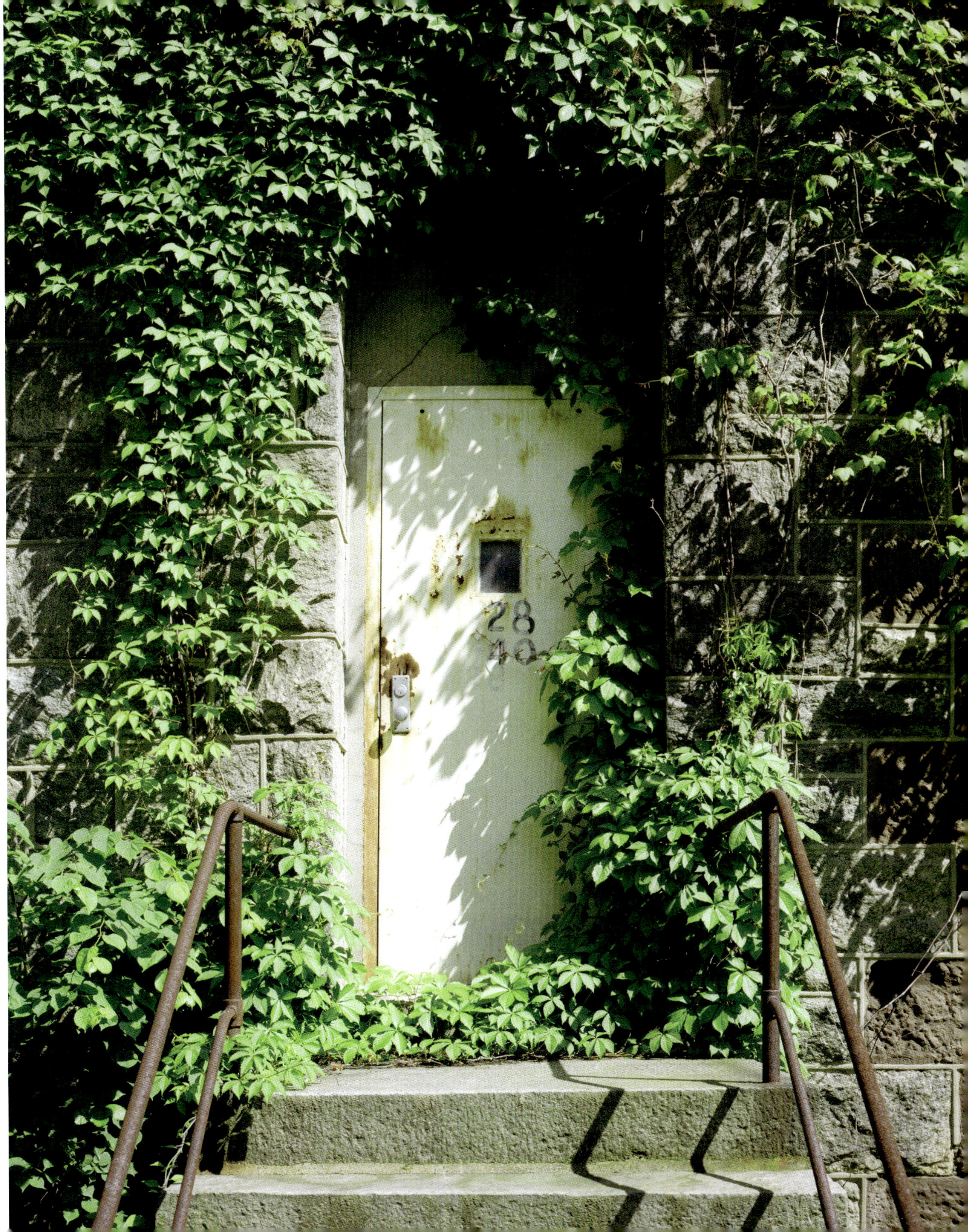
28

She spoke about the importance of a working healthcare system. That's why for her, when she founded the Committee to Combat Huntington's, the issue about public education and information was very important. This had been sort of the dreaded illness–the inherited madness–that went from family member to family member. People kept this totally in the closet. Marjorie wanted to bring this out, to allow people to realize that this is an illness just like any other, for which they hold no blame.

Marjorie was able to empathize with so many people, and served as inspiration for the formation for lay groups in general, for patient-led organizations. There were very few in the mid-1970's, and I think what Marjorie did has been replicated for many diseases. It's different to what was established in other organizations that were focused just on research.–*Dr. Michael Hayden*

When Woody became ill I was told that the case was hopeless and helpless. Assuming that was so, I just said, well, I've got to live with hopeless and helpless. And if my children have the disease, I'm going to have to live with that too.

But after a long period, in and out of that hospital, I said to myself, "Why is it hopeless and helpless?" And with my kids now being old enough to be able to take care of themselves, I went to Dr. Whittier, who was in charge of Creedmoor Institute, where Woody was at that time, and said I want to help. And he introduced me to some other scientists and they said, "You might be able to help if you could just find families. We believe that this disorder is all over the world, it is hidden, families don't even know they have it, and those that do are so ashamed they don't tell anybody because there's a stigma attached." With that kind of help, I began to look for families with this disease and then founded the Committee to Combat Huntington's Disease. We found the disorder was much more prevalent than anybody believed possible.

When I started the Committee, there was a group of very beautiful young people who were writing letters to Woody. Now they were not interested in Huntington's, they're the people who are really keeping Woody's work alive, but maybe they'd like to do something to help me and on that basis I started the Woody Guthrie Foundation. The Foundation has three purposes. The first is to help me with my work in Huntington's. Another is to try to do the kind of things that Woody would have done if he were alive. We just gave a grant to a young woman who's been following the migratory workers around. You know, they're still there. And she's preparing a beautiful photographic essay on child labor and what it's like out in the fields today. And the third goal of the Woody Guthrie Foundation is to get all the material that he left us, all the things I call "The Archives" into some kind of condition so that young people can come to the archives, can read what he wrote, what he stood for, and then go out and write their own things.—*Marjorie Guthrie*

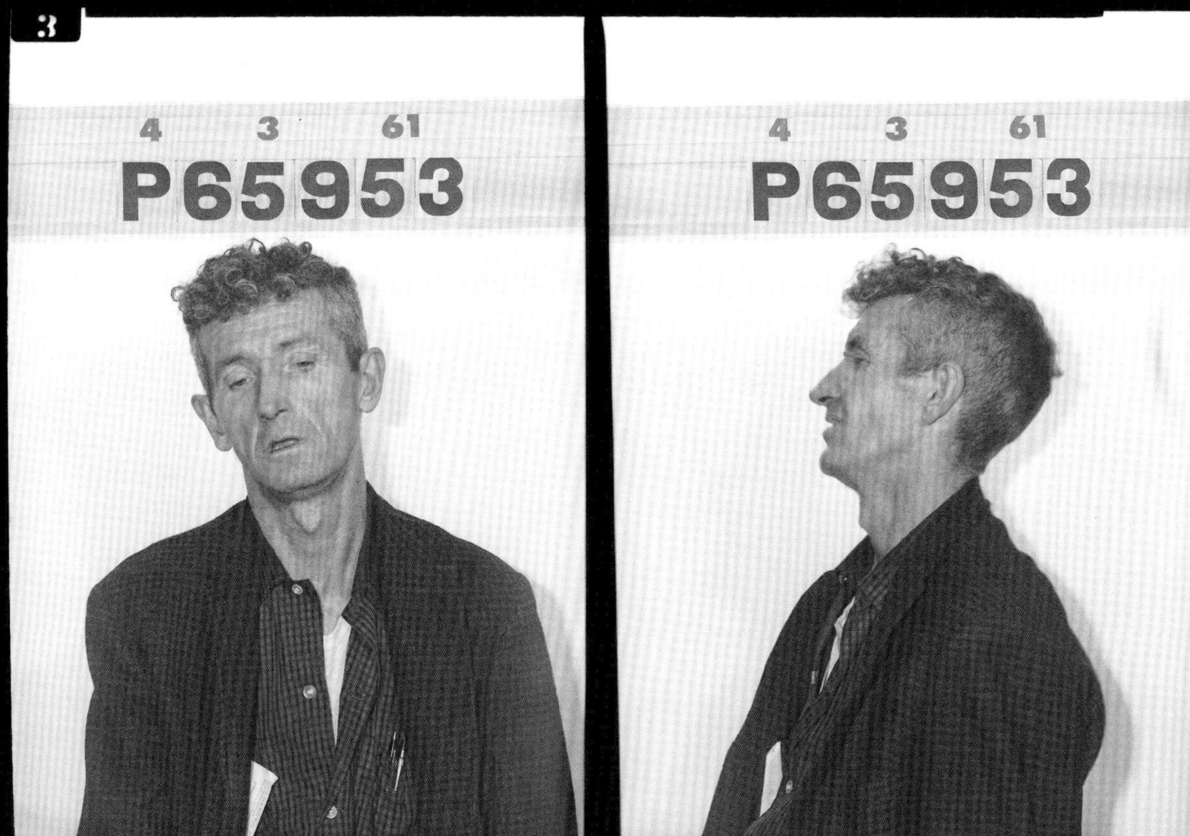
3
4 3 61
P65953
4 3 61
P65953

At the time Woody Guthrie was diagnosed with "Huntington's chorea," as it was called in the 1950s, this disease was known to neurologists but unknown to almost everyone else. Symptoms included involuntary movements (called chorea), cognitive loss, and behavioral disturbances, typically emerging in the thirties or forties and affecting all races and ethnicities. Some families were aware of what they called "the family trouble" or "the shakes" or "St. Vitus's dance," passed down through the generations. But most families didn't talk about it, or tried to deny its existence, for there was no cure, no effective treatment, and sufferers often ended up in mental hospitals. This is what happened to Woody Guthrie's own mother, Nora Belle, who was ultimately institutionalized in Norman, Oklahoma's psychiatric hospital when Woody was nine years old. In his 1943 autobiography Bound For Glory, Woody looked to find an explanation for her dangerously erratic behavior and mood swings: "...the speed and hurry, all of this pound and churn, roar and spin, this staggering yell and nervous scream of our little farm town turning into an Oil and Money Rush, it was too much of a load on my Mother's quieter nerves."

The symptoms associated today with Huntington's disease have actually been around for centuries. Chorea, in fact, was common in children following a bout of rheumatic fever; this chorea was also called St. Vitus's dance. But it was temporary and the affected children usually recovered. However in the early nineteenth century, physicians on both sides of the Atlantic began reporting unusual cases of chorea in older patients who did not recover and whose minds were affected. Moreover their symptoms appeared to run in families. Yet it was not until after 1872, when the young physician George Huntington published a description of the chorea he had observed in certain families in his hometown of East Hampton, Long Island, that "Huntington's chorea" became defined as a distinct disease. Huntington was the first to delineate a specific inheritance pattern for this condition. As he described it, only those who developed the illness were in danger of passing it on to their children; once it failed to appear, it would not reappear in subsequent generations. This was the earliest account of what came to be known as "dominant inheritance" in a human neurological disorder, in which each child of an affected parent runs a 50-50 risk of inheriting the parent's disease.

By the early twentieth century, the simultaneous emergence of modern genetics and of eugenics–an influential scientific and social movement for "better breeding"–helped focus scientific and medical interest in Huntington's chorea around the world. But eugenics also intensified the stigmatization of families with Huntington's by promoting the idea that certain types of people were "unfit" and "defective" and should not have children. For families with clearly hereditary illnesses such as Huntington's, eugenics encouraged secrecy and shame, and made it even more difficult for those affected to learn the facts. Indeed, up through the 1960s, neurologists in the USA typically advised the offspring of a parent with a diagnosis of Huntington's chorea not to have children, or even to get sterilized.

In the late 1960s, HD families began to push for change. Alice Pratt in Texas started the Wills Foundation, the first organization devoted to encouraging research on HD. In 1967, Woody's wife Marjorie Guthrie organized the first national Huntington's advocacy group, the Committee to Combat Huntington's Disease (later the Huntington's Disease Society of America). And Milton Wexler in California started the Hereditary Disease Foundation to stimulate scientific interest in HD and to raise money for research. Five years later Marjorie and Milton, along with a small group of neurologists, helped to bring together several hundred clinicians and scientists from around the world at the landmark 1972 Centennial Symposium on Huntington's Disease. It was at this meeting that many investigators learned, from a Venezuelan physician, about clusters of large families with HD living around the northern shore of Lake Maracaibo. These families were critical to later HD research. Another important step forward occurred in 1976, when the US congress established a Commission for the Control of Huntington's Disease and its Consequences. Headed by Nancy Wexler, along with Marjorie and Milton, the Commission conducted public hearings around the country and formulated an agenda for research, treatment, and public education that put the needs of HD families first.

Social and scientific changes are almost always intertwined. As it happened, in the 1970s the biomedical sciences and especially genetics were in the throes of a revolution. For the first time scientists could manipulate DNA. It had long been known that Huntington's was due to a difference or abnormality in a single gene, passed on generation after generation. With the new technologies, it became possible to "map" the gene itself–to find the precise location on a chromosome of the abnormal gene associated with the disease. That project began in 1980 with the work of David Housman at MIT, James Gusella at Harvard, P. Michael Conneally at Indiana University, and Nancy Wexler, then at the US National Institutes of Health and later at Columbia Medical School. Each year of the project (and for many years after), Nancy led an international group of investigators to visit the Venezuelan HD families, securing crucial clinical and genetic data, and dispensing aid to the families. Within just three years, the team succeeded in identifying a genetic "marker" for HD–a stretch of DNA next door to the genetic abnormality–on chromosome 4.

The 1983 marker discovery inspired widespread exhilaration among HD families (and in the genetics community generally). Besides opening up new ways of mapping genes, it provided the first breakthrough in research on a seemingly hopeless disease. The marker also made possible predictive genetic testing for HD, which began in 1986. Those at 50% risk could now find out whether they were fated to develop symptoms, although not when the symptoms might begin. The marker, however, was not the genetic abnormality itself, which continued to elude investigators. Ten more years of work were required before the "gene hunters"–a collaborative group of nearly one hundred researchers working in the USA, Europe, and Latin America under the leadership of the Hereditary Disease Foundation– finally captured their prey. In this second groundbreaking discovery, they learned that the abnormality consists of a variation in the gene for an important protein now called huntingtin. While everyone has the gene for huntingtin, persons with HD have an expanded stretch of

CAGs–the genetic "recipe" for the amino acid glutamine–at one end of this gene. Too many CAGs in the gene means too many glutamines in the huntingtin protein. Most researchers consider that this extra string of glutamines in the huntingtin protein is the root cause of Huntington's disease.

So far the greatest impact of the gene discovery has been in the laboratory rather than the clinic. But ongoing research has illuminated much about the fundamental mechanisms of the illness and opened up a wide array of promising new approaches for therapies. Researchers are experimenting with methods of turning off, or turning down, the huntingtin gene (known as "gene silencing"). They are identifying "genetic modifiers" that might delay the onset of symptoms, trying to push back the illness into old age or even out of the life span altogether. They are developing ways to protect vulnerable neurons from the poisonous effects of the abnormal protein (called neuroprotective strategies). And they are testing compounds that might be used as drugs to treat or prevent the disease. Indeed, treatments for symptoms have improved considerably since Woody's days, with more effective antidepressants, anti-anxiety and antipsychotic drugs, and medications to reduce irritability, chorea, and sleep disturbances.

Predictive testing has also become much simpler and more accurate since the genetic abnormality associated with the disease was identified, though as of 2012, fewer than 20% of adults at risk in the US have opted to have their DNA tested, for there is still no effective method of prevention. And while it remains complex and costly, a new procedure combining in vitro fertilization with genetic testing (called Preimplantation Genetic Diagnosis or PGD) has enabled some persons at 50% risk and some who know they carry the expanded huntingtin gene to have children yet avoid passing on the disease.

Like many behavioral maladies, Huntington's remains a stigmatized condition. But the Americans with Disabilities Act (ADA) of 1990 and the Genetic Information Nondiscrimination Act (GINA) of 2008 have begun to offer some protections. Courageous HD activists have also done much to challenge the legacy of eugenics and to overcome the burdens of secrecy and shame. They have organized support groups, conferences, education days, summer camps for kids, internet blogs, chat rooms, and websites offering information and social solidarity. TV dramas, movies, mysteries, and even graphic novels feature characters at risk or living with the disease.

There is one arena, however, which has not advanced since Woody's days. Long term care remains a scandal in the United States. Persons living with HD and their loved ones–and all those with chronic neurodegenerative and psychiatric illnesses– still struggle mightily to find appropriate and affordable support and care, at home while they are able, in facilities when they are not. It is said that the measure of any society is the way it treats its most vulnerable members, and persons with HD–their families too– continue to suffer from the lack of supportive services as well as from the disease. In this regard we have a long way to go.
– *Alice Wexler, PhD*

Alice Wexler is a board member of the *Hereditary Disease Foundation*, a Research Scholar at the *UCLA Center for the Study of Women*, and the author of *The Woman Who Walked into the Sea: Huntington's and the Making of a Genetic Disease* (2008), and *Mapping Fate: A Memoir of Family, Risk, and Genetic Research* (1995)

For more information about Huntington's disease please contact:

Hereditary Disease Foundation
3960 Broadway
New York, NY 10032
www.hdfoundation.org

Huntington's Disease Society of America
505 Eighth Avenue, Suite 902
New York, NY 10018
www.hdsa.org

WOODY GUTHRIE

Take it easy. But take it.

Woody Guthrie (1912-1967), one of America's great singer/songwriters, is best known for his folk classic "This Land Is Your Land." His childhood in Oklahoma during the Great Depression and later travels during the Dust Bowl migration gave him a lifelong identification with the common man, and this was one of the factors that made him so approachable to audiences. While Woody was at Greystone Park Hospital, his music was influencing an entire new generation, including Phil Ochs, Bruce Springsteen, John Mellencamp, Joe Strummer, Billy Bragg, Tom Paxton, Ramblin' Jack Elliott and Bob Dylan, who first met Woody at Greystone.

Woody Guthrie would not likely have led the life he did if not for his mother's Huntington's disease. His father was a successful businessman during the Oklahoma oil boom after World War I, but his mother's instability and the Great Depression led to the dissolution of his father's business and their family. Woody wrote about his mother's illness in his 1943 autobiography, *Bound for Glory*:

> *The whole town knew about her. She got careless with her appearance. She let herself run down. She walked around over the town, looking and thinking and crying. The doctor called it insanity and let it go at that. She lost control over the muscles of her face. Us kids would stand around in the house lost in silence, not saying a word for hours, and ashamed, somehow, to go out down the street and play with the kids, and wanting to stay there and see how long her spell would last, and if we could help her. She couldn't control her arms, nor her legs, nor the muscles in her body, and she would go into spasms and fall on the floor, and wallow around through the house, and ruin her clothes, and yell till people blocks up the street could hear her.*
>
> *She would be all right for a while and treat us kids as good as any mother, and all at once it would start in—something bad... and turn into another person, it looked like, standing right there before Roy and me.*

She was sent to an insane asylum after severely burning Woody's father. Woody was fifteen and never saw his mother again. His father moved to Pampa, Texas to live with relatives while he recuperated from his burns. Woody and older brother Roy remained on their own in Okemah for eighteen months before following their father to Pampa. In Pampa, Woody learned to play guitar from his uncle, Jeff Guthrie, and began performing as part of The Corn Cob Trio. But the Great Depression, combined with the Great Dust Storm of 1935, made it difficult to make a living in Texas.

In 1934, at age 22, Woody hitchhiked and rode freight trains to California, as did 400,000 other people during the Dust Bowl migration. Those travels, experiences, and observations about social injustice would later be reflected in the songs Guthrie wrote and performed over the next 15 years.

In the late 1940s, Woody's behavior started to become unpredictable and in 1952, his second wife Marjorie became concerned about his behavior and, for the safety of their children, refused to allow him back into their home. He later voluntarily checked himself into Brooklyn State Hospital, where his Huntington's disease was finally diagnosed in September of 1952. Woody was in and out of Brooklyn State through May of 1956, when he checked himself out and boarded a bus for Philadelphia. He was soon picked up in Morristown, New Jersey, for vagrancy and brought to Greystone Park Psychiatric Hospital, where he was committed after being misdiagnosed as paranoid schizophrenic. There he remained for the next five years.

In 1961, as his health continued to deteriorate, he was transferred to Brooklyn State to be closer to his family. When he could no longer speak, Woody would point to "Yes" or "No" cards that Marjorie would hold. Eventually, he could only communicate by blinking his eyes. He was transferred to Creedmoor Hospital, where a doctor was studying Huntington's disease. Woody died there on October 3, 1967, and his ashes were scattered into the Atlantic Ocean from a jetty in Coney Island.

GREYSTONE PARK STATE HOSPITAL

The last free place in America – Woody Guthrie

The State Asylum for the Insane at Morristown opened in 1877 following the huge need for traumatic care after the Civil War and the efforts of humanitarian activist Dorothea Dix. It was built according to the Kirkbride plan (named for the doctor who developed it) and was considered innovative and enlightened at a time when the mentally ill were often kept in county jails. The Main Building, with 670,000 square feet, is said to have been the largest structure under one roof in the United States until the Pentagon was built in the 1940s. The name was changed to Greystone Park in 1924, after the light-grey gneiss stone used in construction.

Spread over almost 1,000 acres, Greystone was a self-contained community that included staff housing, a post office, fire and police stations, a working farm, vocational and recreational facilities, and its own gas and water utilities. Patients took part in maintaining the grounds and wards, as occupational therapy was one of the few options before the advent of drug treatments. It housed over 6,000 patients and had approximately 2,000 employees at its peak in the 1960s.

Woody was originally housed in Ward 40. Harold Leventhal, Woody's manager, told the author about when he and Fred Hellerman, a member of the blacklisted group The Weavers, came to visit Woody at Greystone. When they asked how he was doing, Woody answered:

> *You don't have to worry about me. I'm worried about how you boys are doing. Out there if you say you're a communist, they'll put you in jail. In here, I can get up there and say I'm a communist and all they'll say is 'Ah, he's crazy.' You know, this is the last free place in America.*

Fifty years after he left, Woody's once-active Ward 40 is in ruin, its fate yet undecided. Many buildings were abandoned following a wide deinstitutionalization of psychiatric patients that began in the mid-1960s. Deemed to be of no historical importance, most of the buildings have been demolished in the past few years, the grounds turned into a county park.

POSTFACE

As I went walking I saw a sign there
And on the sign it said "No Trespassing."
But on the other side it didn't say nothing,
That side was made for you and me.
– Woody Guthrie

My fascination with derelict buildings started with my childhood in a suburban New Jersey town. Exploring ruins was the closest we'd get to feeling like being on an adventure. In 1974, when I was in high school, I rowed to Ellis Island with a friend to make a film about the then-abandoned site. In the 40 years since, I've explored and photographed dozens of ruins. What usually followed was extensive research through archives, online sources, and interviews. Each project now seems to become one of Alice in Wonderland's rabbit holes: I never know what I will find, but I always learn something about myself.

One such project that became much more than I ever imagined began when a friend first suggested Greystone Park Psychiatric Hospital. Hospital memorandums scattered about told that the building had been abandoned in the mid-1970's. There were still traces of life in the corridors and wards, ranging from wheelchairs and beds to ping-pong tables and a shuffleboard court. The asbestos hanging from rusting pipes wasn't as worrisome as the state police station across the street, or whoever might be inside. Coming across the remnants of the hospital's darkroom, it was still full of the patients' intake and discharge photographs. None had names, just case numbers and dates. I wondered about the people for whom Greystone was home.

Later that night after an Internet search, I discovered that Woody Guthrie had been one of those patients. I knew of his role in folk music and that he'd died of a rare disease, but I wasn't all that familiar with his life story or his songs. I began to learn more about Huntington's disease, and that Bob Dylan had traveled to Greystone in 1961 when he was 19 to meet his idol.

I came across a site for the Woody Guthrie Archives and Foundation, which was then located in New York City. Their website (woodyguthrie.org) had a list of material relating to his years at Greystone, including his medical records. I visited the Archives and met Nora Guthrie, Woody's daughter, and showed her some of my photos from Greystone. She and Jorge Arévalo, the head archivist at the time, directed me to letters and more medical records from Woody's time at Greystone. There I found Woody's case number. I headed back to Greystone that week and was surprised to find Woody's photos. His 1956 admittance photo showed a somewhat defiant Woody, but the discharge photo, taken only five years later, saw him looking tired and twenty-five years older. Later that week I gave Nora the negatives for his archives.

I continued to photograph and research for almost ten years, and my explorations at Greystone and the Woody Guthrie Archives would become an art exhibit, incorporating video, photographs, artifacts, music, interviews, and archival documents, which led to this book.

Looking back, I'm amazed at how little I knew of Woody's remarkable life. Listening to a tape of a radio interview with Marjorie Guthrie conducted in 1978, I personally related to how Woody approached his songwriting:

> *Woody never tells people what to do, he tells people what he saw. He never gave answers–he presented the problems.*

I see the book similarly to how I envisioned the art exhibit–I hope you wander back and forth between the pages and make your own personal connections, whether as a fan of Woody's music, as someone who is affected by Huntington's disease, or someone interested in history or historic preservation and the voices we should never stop listening for.

–Phillip Buehler

ACKNOWLEDGMENTS

I am most grateful to Nora Guthrie–without her encouragement, inspiration and boundless enthusiasm and ideas, this book would not have been possible.

Steven Brower's collaboration as designer and editor added an essential layer of beauty and poetry.

In researching Woody's life at Greystone Park, I was especially helped by the Woody Guthrie Archives: Jorge Arévalo, Hillel Arnold, Anna Canoni, Felicia Katz Harris, Michael Smith and Tiffany Collannino, who provided all the archival source captions and credits.

I'd like to thank John Cohen for generously sharing his stories and photographs as well as thoughts on the book. Jeff Carroll, Dr. Vincenzo Cocilovo, Ramblin' Jack Elliott, Arlo Guthrie, Dr. Michael Hayden and Anneke Van Kirk for their stories. And Daye Proffit, son of Bob Gleason, who located Sid Gleason and her husband's photographs. I feel fortunate to have talked with Sid Gleason, Harold Leventhal, and Jim Longhi before they passed away.

To my teachers at the School of Visual Arts, who offered guidance and support for what was first an art installation: Yolanda Cuomo, Marvin Heiferman, Perry Hoberman, Joel Sternfeld and Charles Traub. And Judy McCulloh, for her early support and perspective.

Without Mark Moran or Mark Sceurman, I would never have heard of Greystone. Bill Graef, who accompanied me on those first scary trips to Greystone. Satish Korde and Ed Lebar, who were flexible at my day job. And to many others who offered feedback and encouragement along the way: Jon Birdseye, Tim Blunk, Eddie Elkin, Mark Mocarski, Godfrey Phillips, Peg Schultz, JR Taylor, Steven Wade, Rob Wasserman, Chris Wieliczko, Reven Wurman and Mary Yellin. Danny Frank and Meridian Printing helped make the book look like the original prints.

And finally, I'd like to thank my wife Lisa Levy, my muse who helps me see life as one big art project.

SOURCES, CREDITS AND NOTES: All photographs by Phil Buehler unless otherwise noted.

3. Introduction by Phil Buehler.
5. Leventhal, Harold. Personal interview. 17 March 2004. Leventhal (1919 - 2005) was a music and concert promoter in New York City, Woody Guthrie's manager, and co-founder of the Woody Guthrie Foundation and Archives.
6. The original negative of Guthrie's intake photograph was Woody Guthrie's hospital admission photographs. Greystone Park State Hospital, NJ, June 1956. The original negative of Guthrie's intake photograph was found in the basement of the admissions building by Phil Buehler. Courtesy of Woody Guthrie Archives.
7. Admissions Building.
8. Front Office, Admissions Building.
9. Klein, Joe. Interview with Marjorie Guthrie. 1976 and 1977. Courtesy of the Woody Guthrie Archives.
10. Clinic Building.
11. Woody Guthrie's patient summary, from his Greystone Park State Hospital intake examination. NJ, 29 May 1956. Courtesy of the Woody Guthrie Archives.
12. Cocilovo, Dr. Vincenzo. Personal interview. 1 May 2004. Dr. Cocilovo is a retired physician who was one of Woody's doctors at Greystone Park State Hospital in 1960.
13. Clinic Building.
14. Clinic Building.
15. Excerpt from Woody Guthrie's patient summary, from his Greystone Park State Hospital intake examination. NJ, 29 May 1956. Courtesy of the Woody Guthrie Archives. Photograph by Phil Buehler.
14. Clinic Building.
16. Guthrie, Arlo. Personal interview. 8 October 2002. Guthrie is the son of Woody Guthrie, and a professional musician.
17. Clinic Building.
18. Hayden, Dr. Michael. Personal interview. 14 August 2005 and 11 April 2006. Dr. Hayden is Director and Senior Scientist at the Centre for Molecular Medicine and Therapeutics at the University of British Columbia, Vancouver, Canada where he runs the Hayden Laboratory, focusing on Huntington's genetics research. Dr. Hayden was a friend of Marjorie Guthrie.
19. Admissions Building.
20. Main Building.
21. Ward 40, Main Building.
22. Clinic Building.
23. Guthrie, Arlo. Personal interview. 8 October 2002.
24. Letter to Mrs. Ladlie from Harold Leventhal. Undated.
25. Clinic Building, 1930s postcard, collection of the author.
26. Letter to doctors at Greystone Park State Hospital from Marjorie Guthrie. 18 July 1956. Courtesy of the Woody Guthrie Archives.
27. Clinic Building.
28. "Magiky Tree" in front of Main Building.
29. Clinic Building.
30. Basement level, Cafeteria Building.
31. Clinic Building.
32. Guthrie, Nora "'Life is Tough. You're Lucky If You Live Through It.' Woody Guthrie." (excerpt). 21 April 2006.
33. Woody Guthrie's bed in Ward 18, Clinic Building.
34. Clinic Building.
35. Admissions Building.
36. Letter to Marjorie Guthrie from WoodyGuthrie. 18 August 1956. Courtesy of the Woody Guthrie Archives. Original handwritten letter traced and photographed by Phil Buehler.
37. Admissions Building.
38. Letter to Marjorie Guthrie from Woody Guthrie. Greystone Park State Hospital, NJ, 18 August 1956. Courtesy of the Woody Guthrie Archives. Photograph by Phil Buehler.
39. Recreation Room, Ward 40, Main Building.
40. 360 panorama, Ward 18, Ward 40, Clinic Building.
42. Main Building.
43. Main Building.
44. Corridor with shuffleboard court, Admissions Building.
45. Letter to Nora Guthrie from Woody Guthrie. Greystone Park State Hospital, NJ, 22 October 1956. Guthrie wrote this letter to his daughter across a page filled with domino scores from games played with fellow patients. Courtesy of the Woody Guthrie Archives.
46. Employee Lounge, Cafeteria Building.
47. Ward 18, Clinic Building.
48. Admissions Building.
49. Clinic Building.
50. Hydrotherapy Room, Admissions Building.
51. Letter to Arlo Guthire from Woody Guthrie. Greystone Park State Hospital, NJ, 1956. Courtesy of the Woody Guthrie Archives.
52. Kitchen, Cafeteria Building.
53. Clinic Building.
54. Steam Cabinet, Admissions Building.
55. Service tunnel connecting Admissions Building, Cafeteria Building, and Clinic Building.
56. Letter to Marjorie Guthrie from Woody Guthrie. Greystone Park State Hospital, NJ, 4 October 1956. Courtesy of the Woody Guthrie Archives. Original handwritten letter traced and photographed by Phil Buehler (excerpt).
57. Pharmacy, Clinic Building.
58. Main Building.
59. Letter to Arlo Guthrie from Woody Guthrie. Greystone Park State Hospital, NJ, 1956. Courtesy of the Woody Guthrie Archives. Original handwritten letter traced and photographed by Phil Buehler.
60. Admissions Building.
61. Letter to Nora Guthrie from Woody Guthrie. Greystone Park State Hospital, NJ, 1956. Courtesy of the Woody Guthrie Archives.
62. Leventhal, Harold. Personal interview. 17 March 2004.
63. Harold Leventhal, Woody Guthrie and Lou Gordon. Greystone Park State Hospital, NJ, 1960. Courtesy of Nora Guthrie.
64. Guthrie, Arlo. Personal interview. 8 October 2002.
65. Clinic Building.
66. Gleason, Sidsel. Personal interview. 5 April 2004. Guthrie would often visit family friends Sidsel and her husband, Bob, at their East Orange, NJ home on weekends while he was a patient at Greystone Park State Hospital.
67. Admissions Building.
68. Letter to Nora Guthrie from Woody Guthrie. Greystone Park State Hospital, NJ. 22 October 1956. Courtesy of the Woody Guthrie Archives.
69. Admissions Building.
70. Guthrie, Woody. "The Forsaken Bibel" (excerpt). September 1956. Writing at Greystone Park State Hospital. Courtesy of the Woody Guthrie Archives.
72. Letter to Nora Guthrie from Woody Guthrie. Greystone Park State Hospital, NJ. 15 October 1956. Courtesy of the Woody Guthrie Archives.
73. Admissions Building.
74. Leventhal, Harold. Personal interview. 17 March, 2004.
75. Letter to Marjorie Guthrie from Woody Guthrie. Greystone Park State Hospital, NJ. 19 October 1956. Courtesy of the Woody Guthrie Archives.
76. Panorama, Admissions Building.
78. Admissions Building.
79. Letter to Mary Jo Guthrie Edgmon from Woody Guthrie. Greystone Park State Hospital, NJ, 1956. Courtesy of the Woody Guthrie Archives. Original letter traced and photographed by the author.
80. Letter to Joady Guthrie fromWoody Guthrie. Greystone Park State Hospital, NJ, 1956. Courtesy of the Woody Guthrie Archives. Original handwritten letter traced and photographed by Phil Buehler.
81. Composite photograph of Guthrie family members at Greystone Park State Hospital, 1959 - 2002. Original black and white photograph of Nora, Joady, Arlo, and Woody Guthrie at Greystone Park State Hospital, NJ, 1959 (courtesy of Nora Guthrie), superimposed over color photograph of Greystone Park State Hospital, NJ, 2002. Color photograph and composite photography by Phil Buehler.
82. Klein, Joe. Interview with Marjorie Guthrie. 1976 and 1977. Courtesy of the Woody Guthrie Archives.
83. Joady, Woody and Arlo Guthrie. Greystone Park State Hospital, NJ, 1959. Courtesy of Nora Guthrie.
84. "Magiky Tree," Main Building in background.
85. Klein, Joe. Interview with Marjorie Guthrie. 1976 and 1977. Courtesy of the Woody Guthrie Archives.
86. "Magiky Tree".
87. Arlo, Woody, Nora and Marjorie Guthrie. Greystone Park State Hospital, NJ, 1959. Courtesy of Nora Guthrie.
88. Joady, Woody, Arlo and Nora Guthrie. Greystone Park State Hospital, NJ, 1959. Courtesy of Nora Guthrie.
89. Composite photograph of Guthrie family members at Greystone Park State Hospital, 1959 - 2002. Original black and white photograph of Woody, Joady, and Nora Guthrie at Greystone Park State Hospital, NJ, 1959 (courtesy of Nora Guthrie) superimposed over color photograph of Greystone Park State Hospital, NJ, 2002. Color photograph and composite photography by Phil Buehler.

90. Guthrie, Nora "'Life is Tough. You're Lucky If You Live Through It.' Woody Guthrie." (excerpt). 21 April 2006.
91. Composite photograph of Guthrie family members at Greystone Park State Hospital, 1959 - 2002. Original black and white photograph of Nora, Woody, and Arlo Guthrie at Greystone Park State Hospital, NJ, 1959 (courtesy of Nora Guthrie) superimposed over color photograph of Greystone Park State Hospital, NJ, 2002. Color photograph and composite photography by Phil Buehler.
92. Still images captured from moving image footage filmed at Greystone Park State Hospital, NJ. Courtesy of the Nora Guthrie.
93. Letter to Arlo Guthrie from Woody Guthrie (excerpt). Greystone Park State Hospital, NJ, 1956. Courtesy of the Woody Guthrie Archives. Original handwritten letter traced and photographed by Phil Buehler.
94. Nora Guthrie. Greystone Park State Hospital, NJ, 1959. Courtesy of Nora Guthrie.
95. Guthrie, Arlo. Personal interview. 8 October 2002.
96. Exercise yard, Wards 28 and 40, Main Building.
97. Main entrance, Admissions Building.
98. Letter to Joady Guthrie from Woody Guthrie. Greystone Park State Hospital, NJ, undated. Courtesy of the Woody Guthrie Archives. Photograph by Phil Buehler.
99. Fresco on the wall of Ward 40, Main Building. Signed "W. Courtney."
100. Klein, Joe. Interview with Marjorie Guthrie. 1976 and 1977. Courtesy of the Woody Guthrie Archives.
101. Fresco reproduction of Thomas Hart Benton's "Music Lesson," Ward 40, Main Building.
102. Fresco on the wall of Ward 40, Main Building. Signed "W. Courtney." Copied from John Seuart Curry's "Tornado Over Kansas."
103. Letter to Marjorie Guthrie from Woody Guthrie (excerpt). Greystone Park State Hospital, NJ, 1956. Courtesy of the Woody Guthrie Archives. Original handwritten letter traced and photographed by Phil Buehler.
104. Elkins, Eddie. Interview with Marjorie Guthrie for his radio program on WHRW at the State University of New York. Binghamton, NY, 1978. Courtesy of the Woody Guthrie Archives.
105. Fresco on the wall of Ward 40, Main Building.
106. Ward 40, Main Building. A "lock down" ward where doors have slots for meal trays.
107. Guthrie, Arlo. Personal interview. 8 October 2002.
108. Olesko, Ron. Interview with Marjorie Guthrie for his radio program on WFUV. New York, NY, 1977. Courtesy of Ron Olesko.
109. Gleason, Sidsel. Personal interview. 5 April 2004 and 21 October 2004.
110. Ernie Marrs and Woody Guthrie, 1961. Photographs by Bob Gleason. Courtesy of Sidsel Gleason.
111. Gleason, Sidsel. Personal interview. 5 April 2004 and 21 October 2004.
112. Cohen, John. Personal interview. 11 May 2004 and 14 July 2005. Cohen is a professional photographer, musicologist, and was a founding member of the musical group the New Lost City Ramblers. He was a friend of Woody Guthrie.
113. Sidsel Gleason, John Cohen and Woody Guthrie at the Gleason's home, 1960. Courtesy of John Cohen.
114. Cohen, John. Personal interview. 11 May 2004 and 14 July 2005.
115. Woody Guthrie. Photograph by Bob Gleason. Courtesy of Sidsel Gleason.
116. Ramblin' Jack Elliott and Woody Guthrie. Photographs by and courtesy of John Cohen. Elliott, Ramblin' Jack. Personal interview. 20 September 2004. Elliott is a professional musician, and close family friend of the Guthrie's.
118. Gleason, Sidsel. Personal interview. 5 April 2004 and 21 October 2004.
119. Woody Guthrie's hospital shirt. Courtesy of the Nora Guthrie. Photograph by Phil Buehler.
120. Toshi Seeger and Sidsel Gleason; Ernie Marrs; Pete Seeger and Woody Guthrie at the Seeger's home. Beacon, NY, 1961. Photographs by Bob Gleason. Courtesy of Sidsel Gleason.
121. Gleason, Sidsel. Personal interview. 5 April 2004 and 21 October 2004.
122. "Where Can I Get That Song?" Song index for People's Songs magazine. Photograph of Woody Guthrie by Sid Grossman. Artwork by Woody Guthrie. Courtesy of the Woody Guthrie Archives. Bob Dylan. New York City, NY, 1962. Photograph by and courtesy of John Cohen.
123. "Song to Woody" by Bob Dylan. 14 February 1961. Courtesy of Sidsel Gleason. ©1962, 1990 by Music Corporation of America, Inc. All rights administered by Songs of Universal, Inc. / BMI used by permission. All Rights Reserved.
124. Guthrie, Woody. Bound For Glory. E.P. Dutton, NY, 1943. Courtesy of Sidsel Gleason.
125. Gleason, Sidsel. Personal interview. 5 April 2004 and 21 October 2004.
126. Cohen, John. Personal interview. 11 May 2004 and 14 July 2005.
127. Admissions Building, open window where author first gained entry.
128. Guthrie, Nora "'Life is Tough. You're Lucky If You Live Through It.' Woody Guthrie." (excerpt). 21 April 2006.
129. Admissions Building.
130. Leventhal, Harold. Personal interview. 17 March 2004.
131. Clinic Building.
132. Cohen, John. Personal interview. 11 May 2004 and 14 July 2005.
133. Woody Guthrie. Greystone Park State Hospital, NJ, 1956. Courtesy of the Woody Guthrie Archives. Photograph by Phil Buehler.
134. Woody and Marjorie Guthrie, Howard Beach, New York, 1961, Courtesy of Nora, Guthrie. Guthrie, Nora "'Life is Tough. You're Lucky If You Live Through It.' Woody Guthrie." (excerpt). 21 April 2006.
136. Guthrie, Arlo. Personal interview. 8 October 2002.
137. Letter to Marjorie Guthrie to Woody Guthrie. Greystone Park State Hospital, NJ. 25 October 1956. Courtesy of the Woody Guthrie Archives.
138. Cocilovo, Dr. Vincenzo. Personal interview. 1 May 2004.
139. Woody Guthrie. Courtesy of the Woody Guthrie Archives.
140. Woody Guthrie and Ramblin' Jack Elliott. Gleason family home, East Orange, NJ. Photograph by and courtesy of John Cohen.
141. Elliott, Ramblin' Jack. Personal interview. 20 September 2004.
142. Hayden, Dr. Michael. Personal interview. 14 August 2005 and 11 April 2006.
143. Admissions Building.
144. Leventhal, Harold. Personal interview. 17 March 2004.
145. Admissions Building.
146. Main Building. Guthrie, Marjorie. "A Family Member Speaks about Huntington's Disease. Huntington's Disease." Society of America, 1979.
147. Letter to Marjorie Guthrie from Woody Guthrie. Greystone Park State Hospital, NJ, December 1956. Courtesy of the Woody Guthrie Archives.
"Me you can't even expect it much less ever ask it or demand it. We're done now gone now for real and goney for good and I'm gone forever and for all I feel it's lots lots better now that we are out from each other's hair for all time to come. I hope God lets your labor all succeed as God sees fit and as God sees and as God knows God and but but pray God never let me view thy gloryful [beautes] no more. Peace peace peace peace peace peace. With you and me plumb split off apart. God help me Bye Bye Woody"
148. Operating Room, Clinic Building.
149. Intake/Discharge photograph file room, Admissions Building.
150. Letter to Al Addeo from Woody Guthrie. Greystone Park State Hospital, NJ, 1956. Courtesy of the Woody Guthrie Archives. Photograph by Phil Buehler.
151. Exterior door to exercise yard, Wards 28 and 40, Main Building.
152. Hayden, Dr. Michael. Personal interview. 14 August 2005 and 11 April 2006.
153. Elkins, Eddie. Interview with Marjorie Guthrie for his radio program on WHRW at the State University of New York. Binghamton, NY, 1978. Courtesy of the Woody Guthrie Archives.
155. Woody Guthrie's hospital discharge photographs. Greystone Park State Hospital, NJ, April 4, 1961. The original negative of Guthrie's intake photograph was found in the basement of the admissions building by Phil Buehler. Courtesy of Woody Guthrie Archives.
156. Wexlar, Alice, Ph.D. "A Brief History Of Huntington's Disease." 2011.
158. Buehler, Phillip. "Woody Guthrie: Take it Easy, But Take it."

Front cover: Composite photograph of Guthrie family at Greystone Park State Hospital. Original black and white photograph of Woody, Marjorie, and Nora Guthrie 1959 (courtesy of Nora Guthrie) superimposed over color photograph, 2002, by Phil Buehler.

Back Cover: Courtesy of the Woody Guthrie Archives.

First printed in the United States of America
in 2013 by Woody Guthrie Publications, Inc.
125-131 E. Main Street, Suite #200
Mt. Kisco, NY 10549
www.WoodyGuthrie.org

Photographs and text by Phillip Buehler © 2013 Phillip Buehler
Designed and edited by Steven Brower
Edited by Nora Guthrie
Captions and credits by Anna Canoni and Tiffany Colannino

Cover photograph of Greystone Hospital by Phillip Buehler
Photographs of Woody Guthrie and the Guthrie Family
Courtesy of Nora Guthrie, © Woody Guthrie Publications, Inc.
All writings by Woody Guthrie courtesy of the Woody Guthrie Archives,
© Woody Guthrie Publications, Inc.
Photographs by John Cohen © John Cohen
Photographs by Bob Gleason © Bob Gleason

Printed in the United States of America
Meridian Printing, Rhode Island, USA
Typeset in Hightower

ISBN-10: 0989752100
ISBN-13: 978-0-9897521-0-7

Library of Congress Catalog Control Number: 2013945924